Relax and Enjoy Your Food

Relax and Enjoy Your Food

Save your money, your health, and your sanity by separating fact from flapdoodle

By Craig Good

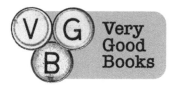

RELAX AND ENJOY YOUR FOOD

Very Good Books

Cover Design by Jeff Pidgeon

Book layout by Alexandru Diaconescu
www.steadfast-typesetting.eu

ISBN-13: 978-1-64062-119-0
Printed and bound in the United States of America

About the book

A lot of people worry about eating the "wrong" food. Well-funded campaigns have spent years convincing you that some foods are good, some are bad, and some are downright evil.

It doesn't have to be that way. *Relax and Enjoy Your Food* uses science and a little common sense to take away all that anxiety, and save you some money to boot. Once you let go of some ideas, it all gets simpler. There are no superfoods, no junk foods, and there aren't even any health foods. There is just food, all of which provides some combination of the same seven basic things that all food does. That's why the most specific advice you can get is to eat a variety of foods, mostly plants, not too much or too little. That's it.

The diet and wellness industries, along with the supplement industry, have deep pockets and ill intent. Their primary victims are women, but everybody gets caught up in their web. After reading this book you'll be able to leave all that behind, eat a healthy diet, even reach and maintain a healthy weight. In short, you'll be able to relax and enjoy your food.

A note about Footnotes

A note about footnotes:

You're holding a paper book. I love you for that. You're going to notice a lot of footnotes are hyperlinks to articles on the web. You're going to think, "Oh, man. I don't want to type all those in."

And then you're going to remember reading this paragraph, telling you that you can find every hyperlink on www.RelaxAndEnjoyYourFood.com, which is a lot less typing.

It will also work for people who listen to the audiobook, of course.

Contents

Introduction

"since the thing perhaps is
to eat flowers and not to be afraid"
— e e cummings,
Complete Poems, 1904–1962

Congratulations on buying this book. Not just because you demonstrated good taste and intelligence. (Or someone you know not only has good taste and intelligence, but also appreciates you enough to gift you a copy.) No matter how you came by it, if you are reading this book then you probably get to choose what you eat. Think about that for a minute. Most of our ancestors ate what they could, when they could. The abundance and variety in today's world is stunning.

You live in the best epoch of all known human history. You are wealthier, healthier, and less likely to die a violent death than most humans who ever lived. The history of our species has been one of starvation, disease, and war. Our ancient ancestors had to make do with whatever food they could scrounge or hunt down and kill. But we did develop something that sets us apart from every other species on the planet.[1] We did it before we even became human. It was such an evolutionary advantage that, arguably, it's why we can afford the big brains we have now. It also freed up time in the day that no longer had to be spent chewing and processing our food.

We are the species that cooks.

As the great apes we are, we evolved in tribes. Cooperation is another one of our great advantages. We can divide up the labor of running our

---

[1] I'm not counting the birds that set fire to grasslands on purpose.

little societies – and now our great ones – and take advantage of agriculture, preparing and cooking food for each other. Cities were invented literally around food. Is it any wonder that food is deeply embedded in every culture? Food isn't just fuel, it's social bonding; the quickest way to a man's heart – and a woman's. It's what mothers provide their children. Food provides us with nourishment and ritual, health and comfort.

Does the name Norman Borlaug ring a bell? It should. In terms of benefit to his fellow man he may be the greatest human who ever lived. Known as the "Father of the Green Revolution",[2] he is credited for saving a billion people from starvation. Yes, a *billion*. Starting in Mexico in the 1940's he developed a high-yield form of wheat that eventually made Mexico a net exporter of wheat. When his work spread to India and Pakistan their wheat yields nearly doubled.

Thanks to advances in modern agriculture you are in the enviable position of not having to scrounge for enough calories to stay alive. You actually get to choose what foods you eat, and how much. Your distant ancestors could scarce dream of the kind of plenty you enjoy, and the myriad flavors you can conjure at the local supermarket or even neighborhood fast food joint.

What a wonderful time to be alive.

So why are you so stressed about what you eat?

Everywhere you turn someone is either shouting the dangers of a certain food or touting the wonders of a super diet. You're warned of "processed foods" and "chemicals" in your diet. Hucksters selling books and nostrums try to convince you your body is awash with "toxins". A massive, multi-billion dollar supplement industry has grown up around distortions and fear tactics, insisting that you must take the right vitamins or minerals to make sure you stay healthy. You're cautioned to buy gluten-free, organic, non-GMO food – that doesn't come from an Industrial Agribusiness. If you don't eat the right berries or leafy greens, well, you may as well be swilling bleach. You're hammered with messages about how the modern food supply is riddled with "silent killers" and is making you sick. Some even tell you that microwave ovens are damaging DNA

---

[2] Scott Kilman and Roger Thurow. "Father of 'Green Revolution' Dies". The Wall Street Journal

or fragile nutrients. You're battered with messages about how much you weigh, or even how much other people weigh. All you know is that you don't weigh the right amount.

It's enough to make you want to pull the blinds and curl up with a bowl of ice cream.

Which is, in a way, exactly what I think you should do. But also with some favorite music and a nice book. This one will do for now.

This is not, by the way, a science book. We aren't going to get into a lot of medical detail. But I've made every effort to make sure that each claim I make is backed up by the current scientific consensus. As it happens, my claims may only sound *heretical* because of the fog of misinformation we all live in.

It's not a weight loss book, either, though it covers pretty much everything you need to know about losing weight. Even if you don't plan on any weight loss, read at least the first part of the chapter *How to Lose Weight Safely* because there are some general cautions there which apply to everybody, and should be of particular interest to parents.

I should take a moment to point out that everything in this book is good news. For you, if not for certain under-regulated industries. I mention it because the reaction I sometimes get to the ideas here is one of anger or disbelief. It's no wonder; some extremely well-funded organizations have spent decades (I'm not kidding) trying to convince you that their view of food and nutrition is the right one. We'll talk about fear-based marketing later in the book. Just wanted to get that out there. So if you feel at any point as though some of your beliefs are being challenged, note that I predicted that. Keep an open mind, roll with the science, and see what you find.

At very least, if you're someone who spends money on supplements, vitamins, or doesn't mind paying a premium for organic food, this book will pay for itself in just a few days. That's pretty good news, isn't it?

The most important thing about your food is your relationship to it. A healthy relationship with food means that making healthy eating choices is trivial. It helps to maintain a healthy weight. It means you never, ever feel guilty about what you eat. It means that you never, ever, need to exercise willpower around food.

Sound liberating?

There's so much hunger out there for good information on food and nutrition. Wouldn't it be nice if there were a simple, no-stress way to eat every day and stay healthy? How much would you like it if you didn't have to think about calories or nutrients and still stay at a healthy weight? How would you like to do all that and save money on your food bill to boot?

There is a way. And you're holding it.

Congratulations.

Chapter 1

Of Fear and Fads

Why me?

You may have noticed that I'm not a scientist, a doctor, or even a nutritionist. So where do I get off writing this book? Well, it has nothing to do with authority or schooling. It does have something to do with years of scientific skepticism, and with my love of food. It has to do with things I learned in the frightening years after my daughter's pediatrician said, "She has *anorexia nervosa*. It has a very high mortality rate." It has to do with what I learned while losing weight. But those aren't the main reason.

Mostly it's because this book needed to be written. It's not that there aren't any other good books on eating, but they're still vastly outnumbered by celebrity-powered codswallop and best-selling flapdoodle. The basic message I want to get across is simple:

Enjoy a variety of foods, mostly plants, including plenty of fruits and vegetables, not too much or too little.

I spent a lot of time on Quora, a question and answer site, answering questions about food and diet. I never had to pretend to know more than I do. None of my thousands of answers relied on any cutting-edge science or required advanced degrees. Yet all of my answers, as all of this book, are grounded in solid science because I do know how to find experts and evaluate claims.

I know not to even claim that I can answer questions outside my knowledge or expertise. The amazing thing to me on Quora was how many times the same simple questions were asked over and over. And over. The amount of confusion and disinformation in the world about food is overwhelming. Confident voices shout from every corner to eat this way or that, avoid this food or the other. Those voices have national television programs, enormously popular web sites, and are fronted by glamorous Hollywood celebrities. Some even have ancient religious traditions behind them.

And most of them are wrong. I'm going to tell you something that they'll almost never tell you: I might be wrong, too.

I've taken every precaution to make sure that, at least at the time of writing, the information I present is scientifically and rationally valid. I convinced experts to fact check the book for me. Even so, just like anybody else, I might be wrong. Being skeptical is the healthiest attitude you can have in life — about everything. I encourage you to follow the footnotes, look at the resources I provide, and seek out the voices of true experts. "Because I said so" is the worst-ever reason to believe something, no matter who says it.

Book Recommendations

I like you already. You read books. That means you won't stop at this one. I'm going to give you some book recommendations, because this book, as marvelous as it is, is not the be-all and end-all. As Ezra Pound said, "Culture begins when one has *forgotten which book*." So bring on the culture. Let's start with a book about food, written by a theologian: *The Gluten Lie: And Other Myths About What You Eat*,[1] by Alan Levinovitz. A theologian, you ask? Yes. Exactly the person to write a book which thoroughly explains where just about every food fad comes from: fear of modernity.

This is exactly the impulse that gave us myths such as Atlantis and the Garden of Eden. It's the notion that long ago things were somehow

---

[1] https://www.amazon.com/Gluten-Lie-Other-Myths-About-ebook/dp/B00T0GIB10/

better, healthier, more natural and peaceful, distinct from the toxic bustle of the present age. Paleo diet, anyone?

Levinovitz can put an exact date on the beginning of the MSG myth:

> The MSG scare began on April 4, 1968, with a letter to the New England Journal of Medicine from Chinese American physician Robert Ho Man Kwok. In the letter, titled "Chinese-Restaurant Syndrome," Kwok reported that after eating in Chinese restaurants he regularly experienced numbness, general weakness, and palpitation. His colleagues had suggested he was allergic to soy sauce, but Kwok knew that couldn't be right. He often used soy sauce in his own home cooking with no ill effect.

Making the classic error of attempting to do science on himself, Kwok incorrectly identified MSG as the culprit, and a scare was born. It's been debunked six ways to Sunday and yet to this day there are people convinced that they're allergic to MSG, or that MSG is somehow not healthful. In fact, MSG is not only harmless but occurs naturally in many foods. Including soy sauce, something Dr. Kwok apparently didn't know. It's a big part of what makes both tomatoes and Parmesan cheese yummy.

The book, as promised by the title, explains that this same fear of modernity led people to think that gluten was somehow bad for them. It's true that for people with Celiac Disease, gluten is a whole lot of bad news. But if you don't happen to have that autoimmune disorder it's simply a nutritious protein that gives baked goods their structure and texture. The logic of thinking that if avoiding gluten is good for Celiacs that it's good for everybody is just like thinking that if crutches are good for people with broken legs then everybody would be better off hobbling around on them.

Levinovitz writes of the Chinese monks, millennia ago, who preached that eating wheat was the root of all evil. Sound familiar? Before and since then, of course, wheat has literally helped build civilization.

As an aside, *The Gluten Lie* not only teaches great lessons on the history of food scares and promotes a healthy relationship with food, it's delightfully well written. I laughed like crazy at the last chapter. No, I won't spoil it for you. Yes, theologian Levinovitz was exactly the right guy to write it.

Because food fears are religious.

Even if you don't need to lose weight, consider reading *Secrets From the Eating Lab: The Science of Weight Loss, the Myth of Willpower, and Why You Should Never Diet Again*[2] by Traci Mann, PhD. Since there's only so much to say about weight loss, much of the book has great tips on modifying your eating habits, and that's something you'll want to do no matter your weight goals.

While it's not about food, I highly recommend that you get a copy of *The Skeptics' Guide to the Universe: How to Know What's Really Real in a World Increasingly Full of Fake*[3] by Dr. Steven Novella. The title kind of says it all. There's so much fake out there about food that the book will equip you to suss out what information is fresh and which is, shall we say, well past its best-by date.

The Orthorexics

You've met orthorexics, though you may not know it. Ortho- comes from the Greek for "straight, upright, rectangular, regular; true, correct, proper," while -rexis means "appetite". Orthorexia was coined in 1997 by physician Steven Bratman. He used it to describe himself.

> "I pursued wellness through healthy eating for years, but grad-ually I began to sense that something was going wrong. The poetry of my life was disappearing. My ability to carry on nor-mal conversations was hindered by intrusive thoughts of food. The need to obtain meals free of meat, fat, and artificial chemicals had put nearly all social forms of eating beyond my reach. I was lonely and obsessed...I found it terribly difficult to free myself. I had been seduced by righteous eating. The problem of my life's meaning had been transferred inexorably to food, and I could not reclaim it."[4]

---

[2] https://www.amazon.com/Secrets-Eating-Lab-Science-Willpower-ebook/dp/B00LSRU7FW/

[3] https://www.amazon.com/Skeptics-Guide-Universe-Really-Increasingly-ebook/dp/B079L5FDBJ/

[4] http://www.orthorexia.com/

It is not yet an actual diagnosis in the DSM,[5] though some day it might be. In this book I'll talk about it as an attitude rather than as a disorder. Raise your hand if someone has told you that if you eat sugar you're poisoning yourself. Or told you to put down that burger and have some kale. Or told you that you need to eat organic, avoid GMOs, shun gluten, get a detox, or add a magical ingredient such as turmeric or coconut oil to your life to reap the amazing health benefits.

You can put your hand down now. You still need at least one to hold the book.

The person who told you all that was in the throes of an orthorexic attitude. They found the way you ate to be un-righteous. Now you can really see why a theologian was the right guy to write that book.

Louise Foxcroft, author of *Calories and Corsets: A History of Dieting Over 2,000 Years*, was interviewed for an episode of the Gastropod podcast.[6] She noted that the ancient Greeks understood that a healthy mind and healthy body made for a healthy society.

> But the ancient Greek influence on diet culture had some built in biases that still resonate today. According to Foxcroft, the ideal body was male. "The male is quite slim, he's quite muscled, and he's very beautiful," she told us. "Women can't live up to that—or weren't thought to be able to live up to that. So the onus on diet and on having an ideal body—it's always been a much more difficult concept for women, and that's reflected in our modern diet culture as well." At the same time, early Christian concepts of gluttony, temptation, and morality condemned fat as sin written on the body—another idea that has shaped Western thought on food and weight for millennia.

Righteous eating indeed. Fervor around the fallacy that "if it's natural it is good" leads many people to think that if it isn't "natural" it must be morally wrong. It appears, for example, that this moral confusion[7] is

---

[5] Diagnostic and Statistical Manual, the book used by the American Psychiatric Association to define mental disorders for diagnosis.

[6] https://gastropod.com/weve-lost-diet-episode-2/

[7] https://www.annualreviews.org/doi/full/10.1146/annurev-nutr-071715-051223

a major part of why much of the public shuns GMOs when nearly all scientists recognize the technology to be extremely safe.

Think about all of those fervent admonitions. At their core every one of them is based in fear. Fear of eating the wrong thing. Fear of not eating the right thing. Fear of eternal punishment. Fear of the modern world.

It's a lot easier to frighten people than to educate them.

Eating is one of the most intimate activities in our lives. Food goes straight into our mouths and passes into the stomach, where it literally becomes a part of us. Of course we're concerned about what we eat! And that makes us vulnerable.

If you remember only one message from this book, I hope it's this one: **Anybody who ever tries to frighten you about a food, an ingredient, or make you feel guilty for how you eat, is someone you should ignore for the rest of your life.**

We're going to examine a lot of these fear techniques and misunderstandings, giving them the skeptical once-over, and relegate them to the compost bin. The last thing you should ever feel about what you eat is guilt. There is nothing on your plate that you need to fear.

Here is how most bad ideas in the world are sold: 1) Invent a problem. 2) Sell the solution. This isn't limited to food and diet, of course; it's extremely common. That web site, fronted by the attractive young woman or celebrity, scares you into being afraid of a food, or of "toxins" in your body, or of how "Big Pharma" or "Big Agriculture" is trying to kill you — and, oh! What's this? They just happen to sell supplements! Or detoxes! Or magical foods! What a coincidence.

The Root of All Fears

I've already mentioned Levinovitz's sage observation that food fads stem from a fear of modernity. While things like anti-GMO panics and the so-called Paleo Diet are obvious examples, fear of the modern world can also manifest as something often called chemophobia. I'll define it as an irrational fear of chemicals or ingredients with scary sounding names.

There's an industrial chemical that is nearly a universal solvent. It's used in a wide variety of products and processes from insecticide to power generation. It can disrupt DNA, is a key component of toxic compounds such as Sulphuric Acid and Nitroglycerin, and is emitted as a large part of automobile exhaust. You're breathing some right now, and there's nothing you can do to prevent it. It's called Dihydrogen Monoxide (DHMO), and it's been known to be fatal to toddlers as well as causing billions of dollars in property damage worldwide every year. That's a pretty scary sounding chemical unless you remember enough high school chemistry or have already visited the brilliant web site, DHMO.org.[8]

Because the common name for this chemical is *water*.

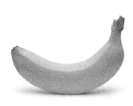

INGREDIENTS: WATER (75%), **SUGARS (12%)** (GLUCOSE (48%), FRUCTOSE (40%), SUCROSE (2%), MALTOSE (<1%)), STARCH (5%), **FIBRE (3%)** (E460, E461, E462, E464, E466, E467) **AMINO ACIDS** (GLUTAMIC ACID (19%), ASPARTIC ACID (16%), HISTIDINE (11%), LEUCINE (7%), LYSINE (5%), PHENYLALANINE (4%), ARGININE (4%), VALINE (4%), ALANINE (4%), SERINE (4%), GLYCINE (3%), THREONINE (3%), ISOLEUCINE (3%), PROLINE (3%), TRYPTOPHAN (1%), CYSTINE (1%), TYROSINE (1%), METHIONINE (1%)), **FATTY ACIDS (1%)** (PALMITIC ACID (30%), OMEGA-6 FATTY ACID: LINOLEIC ACID (14%), OMEGA-3 FATTY ACID: LINOLENIC ACID (8%), OLEIC ACID (7%), PALMITOLEIC ACID (3%), STEARIC ACID (2%), LAURIC ACID (1%), MYRISTIC ACID (1%), CAPRIC ACID (<1%)), ASH (<1%), PHYTOSTEROLS, E515, OXALIC ACID, E300, E306 (TOCOPHEROL), PHYLLOQUINONE, THIAMIN, **COLOURS** (YELLOW-ORANGE E101 (RIBOFLAVIN), YELLOW-BROWN E160a), **FLAVOURS** (ETHYL HEXANOATE, ETHYL BUTANOATE, 3-METHYLBUT-1-YL ETHANOATE, PENTYL ACETATE), E1510, NATURAL RIPENING AGENT (ETHENE GAS).

Image courtesy of James Kennedy[9]

Michael Pollan is a fairly mild example of a chemophobic, what with advising you not eat things you can't pronounce. (As if syllable count affected nutrition.) Vani Hari, the self-styled "Food Babe" is chemophobia's poster child. With a sincerity that can only come from a comically lacking background in chemistry she tries to frighten her "army" into avoiding harmless food ingredients just because they're also used indus-

---

[8] http://www.dhmo.org/facts.html
[9] https://jameskennedymonash.wordpress.com/

trially. It's exactly the same thing I just did with water. For example, she cowed Subway, a major sandwich chain, into removing *azodicarbonamide* (ooh, scary!) from its bread, pounding on her high chair that it's also used in the production of yoga mats. It's true, but it's also true of water. The chemical is perfectly harmless to eat in the amounts that were in the bread. Just because an ingredient in your bread is also used to make yoga mats doesn't mean your bread is full of yoga mat.

In the article that launched her science communication career,[10] Yvette d'Entremont (the "Sci Babe"), an analytical chemist with a background in forensics and toxicology, covers that bit of silliness and also writes:

> Hari's campaign last year against the Starbucks Pumpkin Spice Latte drove me to launch my site (don't fuck with a Bostonian's Pumpkin-Spice Anything). She alleged that the PSL has a "toxic" dose of sugar and two (TWO!!) doses of caramel color level IV in carcinogen class 2b.
>
> The word "toxic" has a meaning, and that is "having the effect of a poison." Anything can be poisonous depending on the dose. Enough water can even be poisonous in the right quantity (and can cause a condition called hyponatremia).
>
> But then, the Food Babe has gone on record to say, "There is just no acceptable level of any chemical to ingest, ever." I wonder if anybody's warned her about good old dihydrogen monoxide?

It's a spicy article. You should read it. She links to the chemical data sheet on sugar. Hard to call it a toxin after that. The point here is, again, to not trust anybody trying to make you afraid of a food or an ingredient. Remember that the amount that someone uses the word toxin is typically inversely proportional to how much chemistry they know. A favorite game is to say something that *sounds* smart but is really stupid, such as "don't eat any ingredient you can't pronounce". Tell you what: I speak Spanish, and people eating "keen-wah" aren't pronouncing *quinoa* right. Doesn't mean they shouldn't eat it. By the way it's kih-NO-ah. So there.

Also, I like quinoa. So there.

[10]https://gawker.com/the-food-babe-blogger-is-full-of-shit-1694902226

Chapter 2

All Food is Healthy

Ask the Right Questions

There are no unhealthy foods, only unhealthy diets.

What you eat today doesn't matter.

Sounds crazy, right? How can you be reading a book about healthy eating that comes right out and says that it doesn't matter what you eat?

Well, that *would* be a little crazy. Good thing that's not what I actually said.

The most common questions about food today take the form, *is [this food] healthy?* Or *which is healthier, [this food] or [that food]?* The problem is that they are the wrong questions.

All *food* is healthy, but all *diets* aren't. If it's a food, it does something good for you. If it didn't, it wouldn't be called food. Any food can be part of a healthy diet. The question you need to ask is *how much of my diet should this food comprise?* As the old saw goes, nobody got fat from one meal, and nobody ever became malnourished for skipping one meal.

Remember that we humans evolved in scarcity. Our hunter-gatherer ancestors had to miss not only meals but days of meals. Our bodies are really good at storing the things they need. It's true that we can't survive more than a few days without water, but everything else is pretty flexible. We're all aware of how extra energy is stored as fat, but not as aware that we have stores of every other nutrient we need that are good for at least days, often longer.

There is no nutrient that you need every day. You can go several days without most, and probably weeks without others.

What you eat *today* doesn't matter. What you eat this *month* does.

The mindset I'm encouraging is a big picture. It's like the difference between weather and climate. Weather is what's happening outside *right now*, and climate is the average of what happens over multiple years. Your diet can handle days of sunshine and rain, even snow. It's your dietary climate that really affects your long term health.

Think about the surface of our planet as we experience it. There are mountains, canyons, hills, valleys. At our human scale some of those can be serious obstacles. Did you know that if you scaled the Earth down to the size of a bowling ball that it would be smoother than a bowling ball? Do you think Neil Armstrong could even see the mountains on Earth from his vantage point on the Moon?

That's the kind of perspective you should have about your diet. Thinking about whether an individual food or ingredient is healthy or not is getting lost in the mountains and valleys. Take the bowling ball view from space and consider your diet as a long-term whole. Fine-tuning and hunting down magical ingredients, or obsessing over every meal isn't going to get you as far as keeping your overall diet and lifestyle healthy and varied.

The Calorie Problem

In biology the Calorie Problem is one every animal has to solve in order to survive: Find enough energy. There are many strategies for solving it. Cats tend to hunt, an energy-intensive activity, and then spend most of their time sleeping. Or napping. Or relaxing. It's a way not to expend many calories. Some snakes take this idea further: they eat an animal nearly as big as they are, then live off of it for a month. Other animals, like hummingbirds, have to keep eating almost all the time because of their energy-intensive lifestyles.

One of the main reasons the panda is going extinct is that it evolved its way into a very narrow, difficult diet. They rely on bamboo for 99% of their nutrition. It's so difficult to extract calories from bamboo that they have to eat 12–38 kg (26–84 pounds) of it every day. When they lose even a little habitat they lose a lot of food supply. This has turned out to be a very precarious solution to the calorie problem. Fortunately for *homo sapiens* we evolved to be able to eat just about anything. In that respect we are very much like pigs. Humans do spectacularly well in all sorts of climates and on all kinds of food. Some call it the See Food Diet: I see food and I eat it. This ability to eat a variety of foods is a great advantage of being human. I know they're cute, but be grateful you aren't a panda.

Since our history as hunter-gatherers is one of scarcity and hunger, punctuated by moments of plenty, our bodies are very adept at storing what we need for good periods of time. We're especially good at storing energy, because you just never know when the next famine will be. (For our distant ancestors the answer was usually "soon".) When your body finds itself with more energy than it needs, it likes to store it as fat. When turned back into energy for your body to use it becomes CO_2 and H_2O. If that combination rings a bell from high school chemistry, it's because those are also the products of combustion when a hydrocarbon (like gasoline) burns. That's why people talk about "burning" calories. It doesn't mean that making your body hotter will reduce your body fat. It just means that your body extracts energy from food in a manner that's a lot like fire.

What is a calorie, anyway?

A calorie, you might not know, is actually a unit of potential energy that comes from an old measure of heat. What we here in America call a Calorie (with a big C) on, say, a food label, is actually a kilocalorie, or kcal. Nutrition labels from Europe are actually labeled in kcal. A calorie is simply the amount of heat required to raise the temperature of 1 gram of water by one degree Celsius under standard pressure.[1] Rather than digress too far into a physics lesson, all we need to know for now is that the more calories there are in your food, the more energy your body can potentially get from that food. It's important to remember that just because a certain food has 100 calories doesn't mean your body is going to end up with exactly 100 calories to burn. A number of factors, including the fiber in the food, will affect how much you actually digest and are

[1] https://en.wikipedia.org/wiki/Calorie

able to use or store. But for our purposes it's close enough. Most of the time.

A calorie really is a calorie, but that doesn't mean that your body processes calories from all foods the same way, or at the same speed, or stores the excess the same way. That part is complicated. But as a matter of physics, a calorie really is a calorie. We'll get into more detail later, but you may want to read what the SciBabe, Yvette D'Entremont has to say on the subject.[2]

Energy isn't the only thing your body can store or do without for the short term. Your requirements are first for oxygen, next for water, and finally food. There's a small list of nutrients that you need in tiny amounts and which your body can't manufacture on its own. Those are known as vitamins and minerals. But your body doesn't run out of them in a day if it has a decent store.

Modern humans in modern nations have not only solved the calorie problem, we've over-solved it. Food is cheap, plentiful, and much of it calorie dense. Outside of the poorest areas on the planet it's just about impossible to starve to death. If you think about it, it's a nice problem to have.

Unfortunately many people now perceive calories as a bad thing. Being overweight is such a common concern that we get bombarded with messages saying calories are unhealthy. Some people even say one food is "healthier" than another because it has fewer calories. But calories aren't bad. Without them we'd die. Ask your caveman ancestor. Or ask a panda.

It's not the what, it's the how much

Paracelsus was one of the pioneers of what would eventually become modern science and medicine. Contrary to medical practitioners of his day, which was the early 1500s, he advocated actually observing nature rather than resorting to ancient texts. One of his observations is still understood to be right today: *The dose is the poison.* He realized that very small amounts of even horrific poisons were harmless, and large doses of apparently benign substances were deadly. And it's true. You can even poison yourself to death by drinking too much water too quickly.

---

[2] https://www.self.com/story/are-all-calories-the-same

We'll get back to Paracelsus and the dose response later. For now I want to point out that it's true for any food: What kind of food it is doesn't matter, but how much of it you eat. That's why I say that all *food* is healthy, but all *diets* aren't. Obsessing over details just isn't helpful. Think big picture. You don't put a lot of thought into exactly where you place each foot, you just generally walk in the right direction.

You can't hurt yourself in one meal. You can't even hurt yourself in one day of eating. In fact, you could probably easily go a week eating just *whatever* and not do anything worse than feel kind of weird for a while.

When you focus on individual meals or, worse, individual ingredients and nutrients, you are thinking about the placement of each foot and the alignment of each toe rather than just enjoying your walk.

Is [this food] healthy?

How many times have you heard that what you were eating wasn't as healthy as something else? One reason that this is the wrong question is that there is no single metric of *healthy* that you can use for comparison. Give me a scale and I can tell you which food is *heavier*. Give me a ruler and I can tell you which food is *taller*. Give me a Bomb Calorimeter and I can probably even tell you how many calories it contains. But there is no instrument that can measure *healthy*.

One of the most common thinking mistakes people make is oversimplification. We like simple answers. If we can stick a label (good/bad) or a number on something then we don't have to think about it much. That's part of why it's tempting to think "calories are bad", or "kale is healthier than cupcakes". But it just doesn't work that way.

Even a cupcake has plenty of nutrients that you can actually use, especially energy. And that kale may have vitamins, minerals, and fiber, but it's hardly giving you any energy at all. Both are contributing to your health, just in different ways.

I can hear your question now. "Are you saying that kale isn't healthier than a cupcake? Are you saying they're the same nutritionally?"

No. I'm not saying either of those things. I'm saying that it's impossible to call one food healthier than another, and that either can be part of a healthy diet. To help illustrate the comparison problem, let's try a hypothetical. I have a table set with a kale salad and a frosted chocolate cupcake. A diabetic enters the room and wisely chooses the salad as the better option. But if a recovering anorexic comes in, the cupcake is far and away the healthier choice. Context matters. Hard and fast rules are useless. Again, don't focus on the individual food, but on the whole diet.

You know what getting too many cupcakes in your diet can do. Did you know that overconsumption of kale (and spinach) can lead to hypothyroidism? Those vegetables contain thiocyanate which, in high concentrations, can interfere with adequate iodine nutrition. The thyroid needs iodine to produce its hormone. Again, you should relax. Unless you've been warned off by your medical doctor you don't have to worry about kale and spinach in normal dietary quantities. The point is that you can get too much of a good thing. More is not always better.

Is this actually food?

It's worth pointing out that not everything that provides nutrition is really a food. I don't mean getting snobby about fast food vs. gourmet cooking. The prime example is alcohol. It does provide some nutrition in the form of calories, but it's really a toxic drug, so I don't count it as a food in our context. As we'll discuss further, the level of toxicity depends on the dose and duration of use.

Fun fact: A toxic dose of alcohol is one that makes you feel drunk. That's why it's called being intoxicated. So, yes, people sometimes literally poison themselves on purpose.

You may have heard that small amounts of alcohol are good for you. Not so fast. It turns out that many of the studies reaching that conclusion are flawed.[3] Other studies about wine may be seeing the effect of one or more non-alcoholic ingredients. (Caution: Resveratrol is overhyped.)[4] Alcohol consumption is also associated with obesity, and new science indicates that it may induce overeating.[5] We'll discuss alcohol's carcinogenic properties a bit later in this chapter. Since there is no health

---

[3] http://www.jsad.com/doi/abs/10.15288/jsad.2016.77.185
[4] https://www.quackwatch.org/01QuackeryRelatedTopics/DSH/resveratrol.html
[5] https://www.nature.com/articles/ncomms14014

benefit to consuming alcohol, but many risks at even moderate levels of consumption, for now it's safe to say that while the risks of small to moderate consumption are low, the less alcohol in your diet, the better.

Variety is the key to a healthy diet.

What is a healthy diet? It's a variety of foods, mostly plants, with plenty of fruits and vegetables, not too much or too little.

That might ring a bell. Michael Pollan, in his famous books, says *Eat food, mostly plants, not too much.* It's pithy. He's a great writer. But his definition of food is ultimately fear-based: Only things your grandmother would recognize as food. He eschews complicated-sounding ingredients. Later I'll detail why that's a problem. He says "not too much" as if excess were the only danger related to quantity. But while eating too much can make you unhealthy and shorten your life in the long run, eating too little can injure and kill you very quickly.

(By the way, the food your grandma ate might not have been all that great. A hundred years ago in America there were some pretty crazy ideas about additives, including treating milk with formaldehyde.)

I stress variety because if you eat a sufficiently varied diet there's little else you have to think about. This is a fantastically liberating idea. These days you hear a lot about what foods to avoid; processed and refined foods are usually near the top of the list. One problem with that is that all food is processed to one degree or another. Cooking is processing. So is chewing. Processing doesn't make food bad. Neither does refining an ingredient.

The biggest problem with many modern diets, particularly in America, is a lack of variety. The majority of people's calories often come from two or three species, with wheat and corn marching at the head of the parade. There's nothing wrong with wheat, and there's nothing wrong with corn. There's a lot wrong with letting any one food dominate your diet.

I'm not going to tell you to avoid any kind of food, because avoidance is based on fear and demonization. I encourage you, on the other hand, to see how many different species you can eat from. That's an easy — and fun — way to get variety into your diet. Dairy products are groovy, but they mostly come from one species. There are only so many different kinds of meat at the store. And a lot of wonderful foods are based primarily on wheat and corn. Variety doesn't mean a cheeseburger one day and a bacon cheeseburger the next.

So if you concentrate on a variety of species, inevitably you find yourself hunting down vegetables and fruits. You knew that was coming, right? We all know we're "supposed to eat our vegetables". Sadly, many people see this as some kind of punishment. It isn't. By the time you finish this book you should be well equipped to play one of the games I love to play at my favorite grocery store (one with a bewilderingly wonderful variety of produce): Pick a vegetable you've never heard of before, and learn how to prepare it. (Hint: you can probably put a little butter on it. No restrictions on the *kinds* of foods you can eat, remember?)

There is no such thing as junk food

This book's goal is to improve your relationship with food. That starts with realizing that there are no bad foods. Some people are quite taken aback by this notion. I've been told that I'm claiming that all foods are the same. That's not the case at all. Of course there are foods which should form a bigger part of your diet than others. Not all foods are the same. But if you're thinking about individual foods you aren't thinking about your diet. The diet is what matters.

When certain foods are demonized, for whatever reason, people are literally claiming that those foods have an evil spirit. A demon. I have good news: There are no demons, in food or otherwise. You can have the ice cream, the burger, the fries, even the candy, and it's not going to hurt you a bit *as long as your overall diet has a healthy variety and proportion.*

As crazy as it sounds to accuse a food of being possessed by evil spirits, that's just the tip of the iceberg.

There is no such thing as health food

Wait! Don't throw the book across the room. Hear me out. Once you realize that any food can be part of a healthy diet, then you have to admit that all food is "health food". Just as you can't demonize certain foods as having evil spirits, neither are there holy foods which convey special "health benefits".

There's just food.

Of course foods are different, and provide different kinds of nutrition. Not all foods should form a big part of your long-term diet. No foods are magically better or healthier or more nutritious. Remember, there isn't a single-axis metric for *nutritious*, either. Perhaps what I should have said was:

There are no superfoods

Sorry, but there aren't. Remember that technique of creating a problem using fear and then selling a solution? That's where all so-called "superfoods" come from. Really, there's just food.

So maybe it's time to look at what food actually is, and does. Food is something that provides nutrition. Don't make the mistake of separating calories from nutrition. Calories are the most important nutrition we get from food. (It's true that we need water more critically, but I think you get the idea.) Energy isn't the *only* thing we need from food. The nutrition we get from food can be broken down into seven basic categories:

1. Carbohydrates
2. Protein
3. Fats
4. Hydration
5. Vitamins
6. Minerals
7. Fiber

Carbohydrates mostly provide food energy. Protein can also provide calories, as well as the amino acids your body uses to make the proteins it needs. Fats are a tremendous energy source, and also provide fats that your body can use directly. (A zero-fat diet would be quite unhealthy.) Hydration, that's water. You're mostly made of water, and the body uses water for just about everything. Vitamins are the chemicals your body needs, in small quantities, that it cannot synthesize for itself. They have to come from your food. The same can be said of minerals, since your body can't make those. Fiber plays its own interesting roles. Sometimes it's a buffer for the absorption of sugars (which are carbohydrates) as in the case of whole fruits. It helps keep things moving along in the colon. And it apparently feeds the micro biome in your gut.

That's really about it. This is what your body uses to function, along with the air you breathe. These are all the "health benefits" of food. Your body will, in its individual way, use (or store) what it needs from these seven categories. There is no specific food that you absolutely need. There are no specific foods that provide unique, specific benefits. They really all just sort into those seven buckets. There's really no reason to make dietary decisions based on claimed "health benefits" at all.

Natural, Schmatural

One of the most successful food marketing campaigns in history has used that formula of creating a fear and offering a solution. It preys on fears of big business and "industrial agriculture" and, rather ironically, became a huge industrial agriculture business. It created a "health halo" leveraging another common fallacy known as the Appeal to Nature.[6] This is the notion that something is good because it's "natural" or bad because it's "unnatural" or "synthetic".

Give it a moment of thought and this is clearly another manifestation of the fear of modernity. If things were healthier in days of yore, it was because they lived "closer to the earth" or "in harmony with nature". New-fangled, complicated-sounding things just aren't natural, so they must be bad. A good way to begin to disabuse ourselves of this notion is to attempt to define "natural".

Maybe it's "things found in nature". Dandy. That's actually a pretty good definition, but it includes a lot of things that are trying to kill you, such as earthquakes, nuclear radiation, and arsenic. There's nothing more natural than getting eaten by a predator. Obviously none of that is what we want from our food.

If we take natural to mean "not made by humans" then we run smack into two problems. The first is that it's not particularly useful to describe

---

[6] https://en.wikipedia.org/wiki/Appeal_to_nature

it in negative terms. The second is that we humans are, like it or not, completely part of nature. We're here for exactly the same reasons that orchids and fireflies are. So, no, it's not really things not made by humans. There's that whiff of fear of modernity again. In the context of food we have to grapple with the fact that pretty much everything in our food supply has been cultivated by humans. Genetic modification of crops and livestock started at the dawn of agriculture.

Take corn, or maize,[7] for example. Before it was domesticated in southern Mexico about 9,000 years ago, it produced one puny cob per plant, only about an inch long. That "natural" corn you buy is the product of human-determined selection. So is corn natural or not?

As it turns out, any time you see the word *natural* on a food label it doesn't mean anything useful. At all. It's just a marketing term. Marketing is practically a science now, and skilled people know how to manipulate the emotions we use when making purchasing decisions. Everything, from the brand name and the package design, to the text on the label, is there to do one thing: Get you to buy.

By using *natural* on the label they have done two things: made you afraid of unnatural things (the competition) and offered you a solution (natural goodness). See how that works? It works so well that a very powerful marketing association has been using a particular marketing term for decades, a word with a manufactured health halo that makes it as mighty as a superhero, able to charge double or sometimes triple the normal price.

Organic.

If you paid attention in your science classes you know that organic means something in chemistry. In that context it refers to chemicals and compounds with carbon atoms. In that world sugar is just as organic as gasoline. To be incandescently clear, that's not the organic we're talking about here. Rather it's the organic label attached (primarily) to food. That's the only kind of organic addressed in this book.

Organic is a marketing term.[8]

Period. It's just a term used to market food, and to do it extremely successfully. Organic food sells sometimes for double or even triple the

[7] https://en.wikipedia.org/wiki/Maize
[8] https://risk-monger.com/2017/08/04/how-organic-is-a-marketing-concept/

price of conventional food. Which price would you rather get if you were a food producer?

And which price would you rather pay as a consumer?

I can see the look on your face. Don't worry, I won't take it personally. Hear me out. You've been told that organic food is healthier for you, better for the environment, and has no pesticides. It turns out that all three of those claims are false. (In parts of Europe the pesticide claim is sort of true. But Europe has a serious anti-science attitude problem when it comes to food. More on that later.)

We're fighting the well-funded, highly motivated, decades-long work by some extremely good marketers here. Lets take a look at those claims in some detail.

When researchers actually look at the health outcomes of organic vs. conventional foods they find pretty much no difference. This is unsurprising because the foods are pretty much identical. A large review[9] of those studies found that—

> The published literature lacks strong evidence that organic foods are significantly more nutritious than conventional foods. Consumption of organic foods may reduce exposure to pesticide residues and antibiotic-resistant bacteria.

You may be thinking, well, what about those pesticide residues? Even if it's the case (and there are no guarantees) there's no evidence that small doses of pesticides are harmful. Remember Paracelsus? It's the dose that makes the poison. In fact, the vast majority of the pesticides that are in your food were produced by the plant itself as a natural defense.[10] Cabbage produces around 46 toxins on its own. Note that the toxins are aimed mostly at bugs, not humans, so cabbage is harmless to us. Still, there's a cheaper way to reduce pesticides in your food. Just wash it. Dr. Steven Novella, writing on *Science Based Medicine*,[11] noted:

[9] http://annals.org/aim/article-abstract/1355685/organic-foods-safer-healthier-than-conventional-alternatives-systematic-review

[10] https://www.acsh.org/news/2017/06/13/9999-pesticides-we-eat-are-produced-plants-themselves-11415

[11] https://sciencebasedmedicine.org/no-health-benefits-from-organic-food/

Even if we take the most pro-organic assumption – that there are more pesticides on conventional produce and that those pesticides have greater negative health effects than organic pesticides, it must still be recognized that simply washing fruits and vegetables effectively reduces pesticide residue. If minimized exposure to pesticide residue is your goal, thoroughly washing your produce is probably the easiest and cheapest way to achieve that end.

A systematic review[12] looked specifically at the nutritional content of organic vs. conventional and concluded:

> On the basis of a systematic review of studies of satisfactory quality, there is no evidence of a difference in nutrient quality between organically and conventionally produced foodstuffs. The small differences in nutrient content detected are biologically plausible and mostly relate to differences in production methods.

By the way, note a study of several common herbicides and their effect on corn: The treated corn was sweeter, and had more protein and beneficial minerals.[13] Yup. The nutritional advantage *can* go to the food treated with pesticides.

The United States Department of Agriculture, or USDA, is in charge of the organic standards. This was another brilliant stroke by the organic marketers. They got their lobbyists to convince the government to make it all official, and the rules defining organic came from solid scientific research, and specify how safe and nutritious the food must be.

Wait.

That's what they *want* you to think. In fact the definition of organic comes from the organic marketing association. Imagine pharmaceutical companies being able to set the rules at the FDA. The organic standard doesn't say a thing about the nutritional content of the food, but only how it's produced.[14]

---

[12] https://www.ncbi.nlm.nih.gov/pubmed/19640946

[13] https://geneticliteracyproject.org/2018/03/07/herbicides-make-sweet-corn-sweeter-and-boost-crops-beneficial-mineral-levels-study-finds/

[14] https://sciencebasedmedicine.org/is-organic-food-more-healthful/

The USDA includes this disclaimer right on the National Organic Program web site:[15]

Our regulations do not address food safety or nutrition.

Certified Organic may not mean better health or nutrition, but at least it's better for the environment, right?

Not so much. While part of the standard claims to support sustainability, organic farmers are hardly the only ones working on that. While sustainability is a laudable goal, there are some serious problems with organic agriculture which are not very green.

Organic farmers do use pesticides. Sometimes lots of them. The regulations simply say that they must be natural pesticides, and not synthetic ones. Uh, oh. There's the n-word again. You can probably guess. Natural in this context has no useful scientific meaning. There's an arbitrary list of pesticides that they consider "good", and all others are off limits. Organic farming often involves more pesticides than conventional because the "natural" pesticides aren't as effective. Many are copper based, and are actually quite a bit more toxic than modern pesticides. Ironically, in Europe where the rather benign glyphosate hit all kinds of regulatory hurdles, the much more toxic copper sulfate favored in much organic farming was approved without a whimper.[16]

A 2013 study[17] looked at nitrates leaching into ground water from both intensive organic and intensive conventional farming.

Surprisingly, intensive organic agriculture relying on solid organic matter, such as composted manure that is implemented in the soil prior to planting as the sole fertilizer, resulted in significant down-leaching of nitrate through the vadose zone to the groundwater. On the other hand, similar intensive agriculture that implemented liquid fertilizer through drip irrigation, as commonly practiced in conventional agriculture, resulted in much lower rates of pollution of the vadose zone and groundwater.

[15] https://www.ams.usda.gov/about-ams/programs-offices/national-organic-program
[16] https://geneticliteracyproject.org/2018/03/20/far-more-toxic-than-glyphosate-copper-sulfate-used-by-organic-and-conventional-farmers-cruises-to-european-reauthorization/
[17] https://www.hydrol-earth-syst-sci.net/18/333/2014/hess-18-333-2014.pdf (PDF)

Setting pesticides aside, there's a potentially more serious environmental threat, namely low yields. A farming method that produces less food per acre needs more acres, making it more resource intensive. A study in Germany[18] looked specifically at the land use issue. It found that while the carbon footprints of organic and conventional were essentially the same, organic used about 40% more land. We are already using about 40% of the Earth's land mass for farming.[19] A major new study in Nature[20], while not about organic farming, addresses land use and its impact on climate. Not only do we need more yield than organic provides just to feed the human population, we need to use the arable land more efficiently in order to reduce our carbon footprint.

Dr. Steve Savage, a plant pathologist, examined the USDA's data on organic land use. Because of the yield shortfalls he observed[21], "To have raised all U.S. crops as organic in 2014 would have required farming of 109 million more acres of land. That is an area equivalent to all the parkland and wildland areas in the lower 48 states, or 1.8 times as much as all the urban land in the nation."

Even if we accepted the more modest 20% land penalty claimed by organic proponents there still would not be enough land.

In other words, if the entire world went organic, millions if not billions of people would have to starve.

It's hard to blame the farmers. Even with the lower yields they can expect a premium of 29–32% on the sale of their crops if they go organic. Customers are willing to pay a hefty premium for organic, which just shows to what extent they've been frightened. That fear is is the direct result of deceptive marketing by Big Organic. A report commissioned by Academics Review[22] kicked over that rock:

> The research findings which follow show that organic food marketers were well informed and repeatedly warned that absent

---

[18] https://www.sciencedirect.com/science/article/pii/S0959652617309666
[19] https://news.nationalgeographic.com/news/2005/12/1209_051209_crops_map.html
[20] https://www.nature.com/articles/s41586-018-0757-z
[21] http://www.learnliberty.org/blog/the-organic-industry-is-a-case-study-in-rent-seeking/
[22] http://academicsreview.org/wp-content/uploads/2014/04/Academics-Review_Organic-Marketing-Report1.pdf (PDF)

consumer food safety concerns about less expensive conventionally grown foods, organic sector sales opportunities would be limited. "If the threats posed by cheaper, conventionally produced
products are removed, then the potential to develop organic
foods will be limited," Kay Hamilton, of Promar International
told attendees at the 1999 Organic Food Conference. Hamilton
added that the potential for growth in the organic market would
be limited if the perceived "threats to safe food production are removed". Also, the "potential to develop the organic market would
be limited" if the sector remains fragmented, consumers are satisfied with food safety and if the furor over genetic modification
dies down.

You read that right. If people aren't afraid of conventional foods and
GMOs then organic sales will decline. And they know it.

Nearly every bad thing you have ever heard about genetic engineering of food is propaganda paid for by the organic industry. Nearly. It
turns out that Putin's Russia[23], unable to compete with America tech-
nologically, has borrowed a page from the organic lobby and started
trashing GMOs. (It's telling that Russia also funds a lot of anti-vaccine
propaganda.) This position can also be traced in part to a crank Russian scientist named Lysenko[24] who gained favor with Stalin and single
handedly wrecked Soviet agriculture with his pseudoscience.

Whether it's from deep-pockets organic propaganda or Russian fake
news, fear mongering about GMO food has resulted in the biggest discon-
nect between scientists and the public at large.[25] Most scientists know
that it's perfectly safe, while far too much of the public is afraid. All for
no good reason.

My purpose here is not to trash organic agriculture. But it's such a
huge example of fear-based food marketing, and is responsible for so
much misinformation, that I have to do a convincing job of knocking the

---

[23] https://geneticliteracyproject.org/2017/06/28/opinion-putins-sock-puppets-russia-
uses-anti-gmo-activists-undermine-crop-biotech-science/

[24] https://theness.com/neurologicablog/index.php/gmos-and-the-revenge-of-
lysenko/

[25] https://sciencebasedmedicine.org/we-still-need-better-communication-on-gmos/

health halo off. There's nothing wrong with organic food *per se*. Sometimes you find organic food that looks prettier or tastes better for some reason. But that reason will always be the other ways the farm is run and never about the fact that it's organic. It's just food. And it's no more "natural" or "healthy" than any other food.

Sugar isn't Cocaine, and Bacon Won't Give You Cancer

Pity poor sugar. If there's any one ingredient getting slammed in the popular press these days, it's sugar. It's especially evil if it's "refined" or "processed". Data have been tortured to paint it "as addictive as cocaine". (It isn't. Never confuse *addictive* with habit *forming*.) Entire books have been written about its vast destructive powers.

Gary Taubes, a persuasive writer with a tendency to overshoot the science in an effort to make a point, spends chapter after chapter in his book, *The Case Against Sugar*, trying to convict. As Dr. Harriet Hall points out, that's the problem: The book is a polemic, not a scientific review.[26] Even Taubes has to admit that the clinical evidence doesn't support his thesis:

> "Research...couldn't establish whether or not sugar was truly the cause of these chronic diseases, or whether people (and the laboratory animals used in the experiments) simply ate too much of the stuff, and so got fat first and sick second."

It's the diet, not the ingredient.

You've probably heard that sugar makes kids hyperactive. That's a myth that just won't seem to die. Plenty of research has been done on the purported link to behavior, and it just ain't so.[27]

Dr. Mark Wolraich, chief of Developmental and Behavioral Pediatrics at Oklahoma University Health Sciences Center, researched sugar's effect on children[28] in the 1990s. Yes, that long ago. He concluded, "Sugar does not appear to affect behavior in children." It's worth looking at why the myth is so persistent. Let me tell you a story about a horse.

[26] https://sciencebasedmedicine.org/gary-taubes-and-the-case-against-sugar/
[27] https://www.livescience.com/55754-does-sugar-make-kids-hyper.html
[28] https://www.livescience.com/55754-does-sugar-make-kids-hyper.html

"Clever Hans" (der Kluge Hans in the original German)[29] was an Orlov Trotter Horse who, in the early 1900s, amazed crowds with his ability to do arithmetic among other intellectual feats. His owner, Wilhelm von Osten could pose an addition question, and Hans would tap his foot on the ground the correct number of times. There was a lot of interest at the time in Animal Cognition, and eventually a government panel, called the Hans Commission, was formed to determine if Hans and von Osten were frauds. Government panel? Oh, yeah. Hans was a big deal.

Through some careful observations and blinding it was found that von Osten was not a fraud! Hans could get the right answer even if someone else asked the questions. But (and you knew there had to be a but) it turned out that Hans got the right answer only if he could see his questioner, and only if the person asking the question knew the right answer.

What was actually happening? As Hans approached the right answer, the person making the query would react with subtle movements. Hans was indeed clever, but not in the way people thought. He was simply able to read his interlocutor and recognize when it was time to stop tapping his hoof. This is now known as the Clever Hans Effect, and resonates even today in animal cognition studies.

The investigating psychologist, Oskar Pfungst, whose debunking didn't prevent von Osten and Hans from a successful and lucrative tour, found that he could play the part of Hans. He'd have a subject stand to his right and concentrate mightily on a number or arithmetic problem. Pfungst would then start tapping with his right hand. Often he noticed "a sudden slight upward jerk of the head" as he approached the right answer. This technique, by the way, is part of how so-called "psychics" do what are called cold readings to this very day.

So what does a perspicacious German horse have to do with kids and birthday cake? Think about how Hans' behavior was changed by cues that people didn't even know they were giving. Now imagine what goes through a kid's mind when mom says, "Not too much of that cake! You know it makes you bank off the walls!" Well, it does now, mom.

---

[29] https://en.wikipedia.org/wiki/Clever_Hans

Part of how the sugar/hyperactivity myth got busted was noting how the hyper behavior evaporated when no adults were around warning of the turbocharging effects of sweets. If you doubt that kids look to the adults in their lives for cues about how to behave, observe a toddler who falls down and then looks around to see if it's worth crying or not.

There's another, even more powerful thing at work here. It is probably the most common and persuasive of all cognitive biases: Confirmation Bias.

Put simply, we tend to accept data which support our preconceived ideas and ignore those which don't. So-called "psychics" depend on it for their livelihood. We remember the hits and forget the misses. Try an experiment. Tell yourself the next time you head to work that people driving black cars are all jerks. They cut people off, tailgate, text while driving, and have offensive haircuts. If you have to drive any significant distance at all I can guarantee that you'll find evidence to back up this assertion.

And you probably won't remember the jerk in the white car who cut you off.

So if you've heard that sugar makes kids go supersonic, that's what you're going to notice at the birthday party. It may not even occur to you that the party itself is responsible for quite a bit of rambunctiousness.

Another common myth about sugar is that it's addictive. It isn't. Oh, we can have sugar cravings, but that's not the same thing. Let the SciBabe lay it out for you:[30]

> But let's get this straight. Sugar is not a drug, nor does it act like one in your system. Studies based on models in rats[31] may support this simple conclusion, but studies in humans are more conclusive and suggest otherwise. A review study[32] published in *Neuroscience & Biobehavioral Reviews* in 2014 aimed to find out if eating patterns were similar to those of addictive behaviors. The study found that though eating *in general* could mimic

---

[30] https://theoutline.com/post/2418/who-s-afraid-of-sugar?zd=3&zi=bi2t2dul
[31] http://journals.lww.com/co-clinicalnutrition/pages/article-viewer.aspx?year=2013&issue=07000&article=00011&type=abstract
[32] https://www.sciencedirect.com/science/article/pii/S0149763414002140

addictive behaviors, it was inappropriate to deem sugar in all its incarnations an addictive substance.

Myths about sugar aren't the only things promulgated by confirmation bias, of course. If a believer "feels better" after eating some organic carrots, guess what's getting the credit.

That old fear of modernity creeps in again when people fret about "processed" or "refined" sugar. What they forget is that, chemically, it's all just sugar. Or, more properly, sugars. Anything you find in an ingredient list that ends with -ose is a sugar: glucose, fructose, sucrose, and even lactose. Once you eat them, your body breaks them all down into glucose. Just sugar.

It makes me chuckle when someone rails against the sucrose in table sugar, but praises the fructose in an apple. They're both just sugar. These same people often laud fructose as the "natural" sugar, but recoil in horror at the idea of any food sweetened with HFCS — High Fructose Corn Syrup. That's just a mixture of glucose and fructose with, you guessed it, extra fructose. Ironically, since it tastes sweeter than sucrose, with HFCS you can theoretically have food taste just as sweet as something with cane sugar, but with less actual sugar.

Even funnier is the "table sugar bad, honey (or agave) good" crowd. Both honey and agave are basically — you can see this coming by now, right? — just sugar. Sure, they have other things in them which provide flavor but, when planning your diet, just treat sugar as sugar.

The World Health Organization which, honestly, sometimes goes a little nutty, has recommended that added sugar form no more than an average of 5% of your daily calorie budget, or TDEE. (More on the Total Daily Energy Expenditure in a later chapter.) For a typical adult that works out very roughly to 25 grams per day. This is not a hard and fast rule. In fact, it's half what their rule of thumb used to be not long ago.

Keep in mind that *added* sugar does not include the many sugars which occur naturally in fruits, vegetables, and dairy products. None of that counts against your daily average of 5%. Note also that this is an average. If you have zero added sugar one day, and treat yourself to 50 grams the next day, don't sweat it. The recommendation isn't because there's anything particularly bad about sugar — because there isn't. But sugar is extremely calorie dense, and very quickly absorbed into the body. Big doses over long periods can lead to obesity and its many comorbid risks. Most people in America and, really, the developed world, get far more added sugar in their diets than they should. I'm not saying you should aim to get as much sugar as this advice allows, just that if you keep your added sugar minimal to nothing on most days then you don't have to sweat treating yourself to that pie or milkshake now and then.

There are a couple of reasons why the WHO doesn't care how much sugar you get from fruits and vegetables, and why you don't have to care much, either. One is that whole fruits and vegetables have a lot of fiber. This acts as a buffer in your stomach, spreading out the amount of time it takes to get the sugar into your bloodstream. There are several metabolic effects of rapid sugar uptake which, if chronic, aren't so good for you. You can splurge now and then with no worries, as long as you aren't diabetic, of course. And that fiber means that the sugar density of the food is low enough that it would be very difficult to get too much sugar that way.

Here's another way to picture that: a glass of orange juice. Not only has all or most of the fiber been left behind when you juice the orange, or any other fruit, but it takes a lot of them to make a glass. It takes about 4 or 5 medium oranges to make a cup of juice. So you get the sugar from that many oranges, but all at once.

There's an important thing to note about sweetened drinks (which include those juices but especially sodas). We evolved to be able to regulate our food intake pretty well using various satiety cues. What we didn't evolve with were drinks that were pretty much just sugar and water. For most of history the sweetest drink kids got was mother's milk, and they were weaned off of that in early childhood. When you chug a sweetened drink a number of things happen. As already mentioned you get a very rapid sugar spike, which can play havoc with your insulin levels. The sneaky thing is that it seems to short-circuit your satiety cues. Even though you've just snarfed a lot of calories worth of food energy, the part of your body that tells you how hungry you are at the next meal seems to get bypassed.

That's a large reason why habitually consuming large quantities of sweetened drinks at an early age can lead to obesity. That long term exposure to high amounts of sugar may not make your kid hyper, but evidence shows that it can habituate them to a high sugar diet. Which means more calories with less satiety, leading to overeating. Most American kids get more sugary snacks than they do fresh fruit. If you read and understand this whole book you'll be keeping more fruits around as snacks and less candy anyway. If kids are getting plenty of fresh fruit and only occasional candy, that's clearly a better situation. Same goes for you, too, mom and dad.

There's no need to panic about sugar, but do be smart about it. Added sugar makes a great treat. It makes a lousy staple. And it's not a toxin. So, woo-hoo! Have all the fruits and veggies you want! As long as you're getting a good variety, you don't even have to think about the sugar.

If sugar gets little Hitler mustaches painted on it, poor bacon wanders around with a "kick me" sign permanently taped to its back. No doubt the fact that it tastes awesome and is loved by millions contributes to the orthorexic zeal behind its condemnation. Many religions like to tout sacrifice as a virtue, and spread the idea that anything enjoyable must be bad for you, while things that are good for you must be somehow unpleasant. This is how people get the notion that exercise is some kind of punishment. (It isn't.) Religious feelings around food reflect that idea, with attitudes that if it tastes good it must be bad for you. Which would pretty much make bacon the devil's candy. Fortunately that's not the case at all.

Remember how I cautioned that the WHO sometimes goes a little nutty? You may remember a study from just a few years ago linking red meat and processed meats to cancer. While the underlying science is OK as far as it goes, the way it got reported was, rather expectedly, sensationalist fear mongering. While bad science reporting is sadly all too common, the WHO could have done a better job.

Let's pause here to note that science is hard, and that science communication is also hard. It's hard to blame scientists for not being good at both. Scientists always couch their answers cautiously, avoiding absolutes, and allowing for possible error. That's their job. But it makes them sound unsure to many average readers.[33] This allows snake oil salesmen, who are

---

[33] https://theness.com/neurologicablog/index.php/communicating-risk-and-

always sure of themselves, to drive a wedge between you and the science. (Pro tip: The more sure someone is about something the more skeptical you should be.) Poorly trained journalists don't help much either.

Let's put the study into perspective.[34] They looked at red meat, namely meat from mammals, such as beef, pork and lamb. While they found only limited evidence that high levels of red meat consumption were linked with colorectal cancer, they found a "mechanistic link". All that means is that a link is plausible. For processed meat, meaning salted, cured, or smoked, such as bacon, ham, and jerky, they found an association with colorectal cancer, but never mentioned a mechanism.

According to the study, if you eat about 2 strips of bacon every day, year in and year out, your risk of colorectal cancer goes up by 18%. Ooh, that sounds scary, right? First off, you aren't getting enough variety points if you eat that much bacon every single day. I mean, I love bacon, but that's a lot. The real rub, though, is that 18% is the *relative* risk.

If you eat no meats at all your lifetime risk for colorectal cancer is about 6%. If you chow down on your two strips per day for your whole life then your risk does indeed go up about 18% – to 7%. Yes, you read that right. No meat: 6%. Lots of bacon: 7%. That's the *absolute* risk. Whenever you see percent risk in a news story, find out (if you can) whether it's relative or absolute. That's a distinction that makes a difference.

There were other problems with that study, including that it was an observational study, meaning it's open to all kinds of confounders. Consider the 2009 study[35] that found:

> "Subjects who consumed more red meat tended to be married, more likely to be of non-Hispanic white ethnicity, more likely to be a current smoker, have a higher body mass index, and a higher daily intake of energy, total fat and saturated fat; whereas they tended to have a lower education level, were less physically active and consumed less fruits, vegetables, fiber and vitamin supplements."

[34]https://theness.com/neurologicablog/index.php/who-report-on-red-and-processed-meat/
[35]http://www.ncbi.nlm.nih.gov/pmc/articles/PMC2803089/?tool=pubmed

So the consumption of red meat correlates with other behaviors that could well contribute to a cancer risk. Like smoking. There's no way, in other words, to blame red meat for the entire difference in cancer risk. And it's not at all clear that going vegetarian makes that much difference to this risk. There was a meta-analysis in 2008[36] which found:

> …no significant differences in the mortality caused by colorectal, stomach, lung, prostate or breast cancers and stroke between vegetarians and "health-conscious" nonvegetarians.

Now, it's true that you could even further reduce your cancer risk by switching to nitrite-free cured meats. Genuine Prosciutto di Parma has been that way since 1993, for example. Since it takes a lot longer to cure meat with just salt, expect any such bacon to come at a premium price.

A Side Course of Science

This is a good time to talk about how to consume science news. Consider the following three headlines, all for stories reporting on exactly the same study:

MDLinx: "Bacon, soda and too few nuts tied to big portion of US deaths."

USNews: "Poor Diet Tied to Half of U.S. Deaths from Heart Disease, Diabetes."

Reuters: "Poor diet tied to nearly half of U.S. deaths from heart disease, stroke, diabetes."

Want to take a guess which headline is the most accurate? If you guessed the least sensational, the one from Reuters, treat yourself to a bacon maple donut. But the only way to find out, often is to track down the original paper[37] and read what it actually says. You'd think that journalists would do that, it kind of being their job and everything, but they rarely do. Mostly they're under-trained and overextended, so they take the easy way out. Also, sensational headlines get clicks. Fortunately there are trusted sources of information, such as Science Based Medicine,

---

[36] http://www.ncbi.nlm.nih.gov/pubmed/19166134
[37] http://jamanetwork.com/journals/jama/article-abstract/2608221

where experts who understand scientific papers can sort them out for us.[38]

It's true that the CDC has estimated that nearly half of U.S. deaths could be prevented with lifestyle changes[39], but those changes include not only diet but things like quitting smoking and taking up regular exercise.

But back to that study which produced three different headlines. They studied 10 specific dietary factors, looking for an association with mortality due to heart disease, stroke, and type 2 diabetes. Dr. Harriet Hall, writing in Science Based Medicine, notes:

> They studied fruits, vegetables, nuts/seeds, whole grains, un-processed red meats, processed meats, sugar-sweetened beverages, polyunsaturated fats, seafood omega-3 fats, and sodium. They chose not to study several other dietary factors (monoun-saturated fats, vitamin D, magnesium, calcium, antioxidant vitamins, dairy products, cocoa, coffee, and tea) because of insufficient evidence for a causal relationship. They looked only at cardiometabolic conditions, not at other conditions like cancer, osteoporosis, gallstones, inflammatory diseases, depression, cognitive function, or micronutrient deficiencies.

And did they actually find that eating bacon and too few nuts killed you? Nope. The study is interesting and useful, and did find associations between high consumption levels of some of those foods and increased CMD, or cardiometabolic deaths. By now it should not be surprising that science found that you should eat a variety of things and not too much of any of them. But there are subtleties here. As good scientists, the authors pointed out some potential weaknesses of their own study:

1. Evidence from observational studies is subject to pitfalls and con-founders.
2. We don't know whether the 10 selected factors comprise the right set.

---

[38] https://sciencebasedmedicine.org/dietary-associations-with-cardiovascular-and-diabetic-mortality-bacon-soda-and-too-few-nuts/
[39] http://time.com/84514/nearly-half-of-us-deaths-can-be-prevented-with-lifestyle-changes/

3. Dietary factors are interrelated and modified by each other.

Dr. Hall cautions further:

> Whatever the actual numbers, they undeniably showed that bet-
> ter diet quality (with reference to the 10 items studied) is asso-
> ciated with fewer cardiometabolic deaths. What they did not
> show was that you could take people with poor diet quality and
> reduce their death rate by improving the quality of their diet. It
> might seem intuitively obvious that that would work, but even
> the most compelling assumptions can be wrong. The history
> of science has taught us not to assume but to test. Hypotheses
> about interventions remain to be tested, and will require further
> studies.

Setting cancer aside, meat consumption does associate with increased
risk of heart disease but, again, only at high consumption levels. Once
again, the evidence shows that enjoying a variety of foods, *mostly* plants,
with plenty of fruits and veggies, not too much or too little, is the best
advice.

Don't fret about cancer and food in any case. It won't help, and
it might just damage your healthy relationship with food. Here's why:
Everything we eat causes cancer.[40] Well, sort of. Let me explain.

Studying cancer is complicated. For ethical reasons we can't make
people into guinea pigs for a particular cancer-related variable. So there
are no random, double-blind, placebo-controlled studies. That means
that statistical, longitudinal studies have to carry the freight. Over a long
time, given enough information, probabilities can be teased out of the
data. The links between smoking tobacco and both heart and lung disease
were clearly established by very strong signals in the data using these
kinds of studies. Still, it's not correct to say that smoking *will* give you
cancer. It's more correct to say that it *greatly and significantly increases
your risk* of cancer. The signal is so strong that the scientific consensus for
decades has been *don't smoke*. That consensus is so solid that it's virtually
impossible that science will ever switch to a pro-smoking position.

---

[40]https://sciencebasedmedicine.org/everything-we-eat-causes-cancer/

When it comes to food, there are no signals that strong. That's why we get results like I already mentioned for bacon. In a later chapter we'll talk more about individual studies vs. systematic reviews. For now let's just say that systematic reviews, known as meta-analyses, get you closer to a consensus than any one study does, because they're studies of studies.

Jonathan D. Schoenfeld and John Ioannidis undertook one called *Is everything we eat associated with cancer? A systematic cookbook review.*[41] Instead of reviewing scientific studies, they looked at several cookbook recipes chosen at random and selected 50 common ingredients. Then they searched the scientific literature on cancer risk for occurrences of those ingredients — either as being potentially carcinogenic or potentially lowering cancer risk. By this point you may not even be surprised at what they found.

For 80% of the ingredients there were studies reporting on their cancer risk. 72% found that the ingredient was associated with an increased cancer risk. But 75% of the studies had weak or no statistical significance. For many of the ingredients there were about as many studies claiming an *increased* cancer risk as a *decreased* cancer risk. Even the ingredients (such as bacon) where most or all of the studies showed an increase, the studies had very weak results.

Enter our hero, the meta-analysis. By combining hundreds of individual studies a more accurate picture can emerge. Not surprisingly, the effect sizes all got smaller in the meta-analyses that were combined in this meta-analysis. Yes, this study of studies includes studies of studies. It's like *Inception* or something. Again, this is generally how you get closer to a consensus.

The authors summed up their paper thus:

> Associations with cancer risk or benefits have been claimed for most food ingredients. Many single studies highlight implausibly large effects, even though evidence is weak. Effect sizes shrink in meta-analyses.

This does not mean, to be clear, that you can just ignore every warning you hear, as long as they come from scientists. As summed up by surgical oncologist Dr. David Gorski writing on *Science Based Medicine*:

---

[41] https://www.ncbi.nlm.nih.gov/pubmed/23193004

Indeed, as was pointed out at Cancer Research UK, the real issue is that individual studies taken in isolation can be profoundly misleading. There's so much noise and so many confounders to account for that any single study can easily miss the mark, either overestimating or underestimating associations. Given publication bias and the tendency to believe that some foods or environmental factors must cause cancer, it's not too surprising that studies tend to overestimate effect sizes more often then they underestimate them. Looking through all the noise and trying to find the true signals, there are at least a few foods that are reliably linked to cancer. For instance, alcohol consumption is positively linked with several cancers, including pancreatic, esophageal, and head and neck cancers, among others. There's evidence that eating lots of fruit and vegetables compared to meat can have protective effects against colorectal cancer and others, although the links are not strong, and processed meats like bacon have been linked to various cancers, although, again, the elevated risk is not huge. *When you boil it all down, it's probably far less important what individual foods one eats than that one eats a varied diet that is relatively low in red meat and high in vegetables and fruits and that one is not obese.* (Emphasis added)

While a healthy diet can reduce your risk of cancer, it's important to note that **you cannot prevent or treat cancer with diet**. The idea that people get cancer because they ate the wrong food is wrong-headed victim blaming of a disgusting flavor. The truth is that cancer is often nature's reward for living a very long life. More people die of cancer now because people live longer lives now. And when someone gets cancer it is impossible to say exactly what caused that cancer. Thanks to epidemiology we can say what the most likely contributing factors (such as smoking, alcohol, etc.) were, but the exact cause is unknowable.

Anybody, doctor or not, who tries to sell you on the idea that you can treat your cancer with diet is waddling toward a pond, water rolling off their back. Scammers, cranks, and even well-meaning non-scientists will try to convince you of it. And smart people do get fooled. Even Steve Jobs most likely shortened his life by relying too long on diet to treat his cancer. Cancer is understandably terrifying. Merely being smart isn't enough. That leaves the door open for crazy ideas such as cutting out sugar to "starve" a cancer.

The wife of a friend of mine recently received a cancer diagnosis. That's already a stressful, difficult thing to deal with. But she's being tormented by people piping up with "helpful advice" about what foods to eat to fight off the cancer. Please don't be that "helpful" person who piles harmful stress on top of an already difficult situation.

I repeat: **cancer cannot be treated by diet**. Don't tell your friends who have cancer what they should eat or do. They have doctors for that.

Don't Fear the GMO

Because there is so much irrational fear about the genetic engineering of food, I have to dedicate a whole section of the book to it. The orthorexics, organic marketers, (and Putin), have spent so many millions of dollars to prey on our fears of modernity that it's little wonder that people are afraid of it.

Unfortunately the term GMO, or Genetically Modified Organism, doesn't even make much sense. Every living thing is genetically modified. That's how evolution works. As I mentioned before, pretty much everything we eat has been genetically modified one way or another. We have been genetically modifying our food for thousands of years.[42] Selective breeding has been the longest used method. It's very slow and rather imprecise, but it's gotten us to the corn that we have now.

Mutagenesis[43] is another method used to get newer and better crops. It dates back just about a hundred years now, and essentially uses some kind of stress to force mutations. The first stressor tried was heat, but now both chemical agents and radiation are used as well. Most mutations don't work at all. Researchers are happy to have something useful turn up every now and then. This is a little like smashing windows on the sidewalk and hoping for the right shaped glass shards for your art

---

[42] https://geneticliteracyproject.org/2018/03/02/viewpoint-humans-genetically-modifying-food-thousands-years/

[43] https://en.wikipedia.org/wiki/Mutagenesis

project. It works eventually, but you end up with a lot of unusable glass and a messy sidewalk. Transgenic gene modification, or gene editing (often called GE), is the technology usually misnamed GM. Very precise, targeted, well-understood changes can be made, sometimes borrowing bits of DNA from a different species.

Orthorexic technophobes at this point are recoiling in horror. "Franken-food!" they howl. "Fishmato!" they keen.

So let's agree right now to keep this a secret: Lateral gene transfer, from one species to another, happens all the time in nature. Yeah. GM technology is doing something entirely natural, except it's very exact. It's using a precision glass cutter to get exactly the pieces we want for that art project. Oh, and there's no such thing as a "fishmato". The idea of borrowing some fish DNA to improve tomatoes was a lab experiment. But it's really incorrect to call it "fish DNA". DNA is just DNA, and most life shares a lot of it in common. Forget about other apes; you and the banana in your kitchen share about 50% of your DNA. So does the banana have human DNA? Do you have banana DNA? (To be fair, there are some people I strongly suspect of having quite a bit of banana DNA.) Of course neither is the case. There is just DNA. A gene from a fish isn't a fish gene, it's just a gene that a fish has.

By the way, as of the writing of this book in 2020, there are exactly zero GMO tomatoes on the market. None.

Those well-heeled fear mongers like to claim that GMOs aren't natural. Well, as we already saw, "natural" isn't a very meaningful term, and gene transfer happens all the time in nature anyway. They also claim that it's "untested" or "risky". Neither claim is even in the same Zip Code with the truth.

Among scientists there's no controversy about GMO safety. A shockingly similar science-denial situation to Climate Change deniers exists among anti-GMO zealots. Seriously. The arguments are almost identical: It's a big conspiracy, we can't trust the scientists, we don't have to believe the data, yada yada.

Over the last two decades there have been at least 3,000 studies on GMO safety by around 280 scientific institutions on multiple continents. There have been many long-term studies,[44] and the only reason they

---

[44] https://geneticliteracyproject.org/2017/07/07/true-no-long-term-gmo-safety-

don't go back more than about three decades is that the first GE crop didn't happen until 1982. The overwhelming scientific consensus is that GMO crops are both safe and beneficial.

The difference between scientific opinion and public opinion is, sadly, a chasm when it comes to GMOs. A 2018 Pew study found Americans split roughly 50/50, even though scientists have a favorable view of nearly 100%. Among scientists there is no controversy, but the FUD[45] (Fear, Uncertainty, and Doubt) spread by green and organic propaganda creates the illusion of one. Steven Novella analyzed the results[46] and noted:

> …to quickly summarize: GMOs have not been linked to nega-tive health outcomes, and there are thousands of studies looking at GMOs, more than half of which are independently funded. Use of GMOs has not been linked to Indian farmer suicide. Mon-santo did not sue any farmers over accidental contamination, and never marketed a terminator seed. Farmers don't save their seeds anyway, and you cannot save and replant hybrid seeds (which are most of the non-GMO crops). Not all GMOs are patented, and many non-GMO crops are patented (such as most hybrid breeds). Use of GMOs has actually decreased insecticide use, and has allowed the use of less toxic herbicides. Use of GMOs correlates with higher overall yields and increased profits for farmers. There have been no GMOs on the market that have caused allergies or new toxicity.

One of the greatest benefits to the majority of GE crops is yield. When you get more food out of the same acre of land, it's better for the environment. And many such crops use both fewer pesticides than conventional, and less toxic pesticides. Remember how plants produce their own pesticides? Genetic engineering allows borrowing the ability to produce actually natural pesticides from one plant and install it in another. Plants can also be made resistant to a pesticide that eliminates weeds. That's how the much-maligned glyphosate, some of which is marketed as Round-Up, works. It's not only low in toxicity, but rapidly breaks down into

studies/

45 Fear, Uncertainty, and Doubt

46 https://theness.com/neurologicablog/index.php/new-pew-survey-about-gmos/

harmless components in the soil. While it's toxic to noxious plants, it chemically can't do much of anything to people, which is why it's slightly less toxic to humans than table salt is. Honestly, it's one of the most environmentally responsible pesticides on the market. But admitting that it works would violate the cherished beliefs of anti-GMO science deniers, not to mention take a bite out of Big Organic's market.

A couple of apparently spectacular studies showing the dangers of GMOs got a lot of press a few years ago. A particularly infamous example was the rat study done by anti-GMO activist Gilles-Éric Séralini.[47] It purported to show that GMO corn caused cancer in rats. Real scientists raised such a stink that the paper was eventually retracted,[48] meaning it is no longer considered part of the scientific literature. Setting aside the ethics of how he actually abused the rats in that experiment, it was an example of scientific fraud reminiscent of the kind of bad science produced by anti-vaccine activists. It's not the only anti-GMO paper that's had to be retracted due to scientific fraud.[49] An experiment supposedly showing how GMO corn feed turned pigs' guts to mush was actually an unscientific "fishing expedition", meaning they fed conventional corn to one group, GM corn to another, and then dissected the pigs to hunt for anomalies.[50] Ask the next scientist you meet what kind of science that is. Expect colorful language.

GMOs can not only increase yields, but add vital nutrients to food. In developing parts of the world this can literally be a life saver. A prime example is Golden Rice, engineered to add beta-carotene, a precursor to Vitamin A, to a staple food. It's estimated that it could save the lives of two million children per year. Yet ideologically motivated activists such as Greenpeace are actually on record as preferring dead or blind children to letting farmers plant a GMO crop.[51] That's fear of modernity at its worst.

---

[47] https://geneticliteracyproject.org/glp-facts/gilles-eric-seralini-activist-professor-face-anti-gmo-industry/

[48] https://sciencebasedmedicine.org/the-seralini-gmo-study-retraction-and-response-to-critics/

[49] https://sciencebasedmedicine.org/another-anti-gmo-paper-retracted/

[50] https://sciencebasedmedicine.org/once-more-bad-science-in-the-service-of-anti-gmo-activism/

[51] http://www.independent.co.uk/news/science/former-greenpeace-leading-light-condemns-them-for-opposing-gm-golden-rice-crop-that-could-save-two-9097170.html

Anti-GMO campaigning has a disturbingly racist and classist edge. Almost everybody buying the organic marketing line about the dangers of GMOs is wealthy, healthy, and utterly unconcerned about the distant, poor, mostly brown people who are directly affected when denied the benefits of improved agriculture. In Europe much of the anti-GMO campaigning is ostensibly about "health concerns" but is really motivated by protecting European agriculture from American competition. One net result of European and American anti-GMO policies and scare tactics is that it's killing Africans. One study looked at merely the delay in approving GE crops for small African farms[52]:

> The costs of a delay can be substantial: e.g. a one year delay in approval of the pod-borer resistant cowpea in Nigeria will cost the country about 33 million USD to 46 million USD and between 100 and 3,000 lives.

The funny part is that even organic farmers benefit from GMO crops being grown nearby.[53] Bt GMOs (Bt is a kind of natural pesticide produced by plants, harmless to humans but rough on bugs) not only reduce pesticide use and increase yields, but the "halo effect" of reducing pest populations actually helps the yields of neighboring "organic" farms. A study of Bt Corn, which has safely been grown and consumed since 1996, found that it reduced spraying and crop damage, and helped out neighboring crops.[54]

Pretty much everything the pro-organic, anti-GMO crowd tells you is the reverse of the truth.[55] In fact, a very good case can be made that real environmentalists will favor GMO technology just because its better for the environment.[56]

---

[52] http://journals.plos.org/plosone/article?id=10.1371/journal.pone.0181353

[53] https://thelogicofscience.com/2018/03/20/bt-gmos-reduce-pesticides-increase-yields-and-benefit-farmers-including-organic-farmers/

[54] https://geneticliteracyproject.org/2018/03/13/40-years-of-data-show-bt-corn-significantly-reduces-pests-spraying-and-crop-damage-including-in-nearby-non-gmo-fields/

[55] https://futurism.com/organic-gmo-food-myths/

[56] https://www.forbes.com/sites/omribenshahar/2018/02/26/the-environmentalist-case-in-favor-of-gmo-food/#13a6c90137de

Fear of modernity, and it's ugly twin the Appeal to Nature Fallacy, are powerful weapons. It is much easier to frighten people than to educate them. Many good people have been driven to a fanatical, religious, ideological attitude about their food.[57] And who can blame them? Some very well-funded people have worked very hard for decades to get them there.

Fortunately you, dear reader, have an open mind and the disposition to be healthy, happy, and save money all at the same time. When you stroll through the produce section or food aisles and see "natural", organic, or GMO-free on a label you know what it really says: *We want to frighten you into buying our product, and we think you'll pay extra for it.*

Looking at evidence and listening to experts is how Nobel Laureate Richard Roberts became a GMO advocate.[58]

I was invited to a symposium celebrating Marc Van Montagu's birthday. He's one of the people who discovered how to genetically modify plants using the Agrobacterium system. I spent a day in Ghent at a meeting listening, for the most part, to plant scientists talk about, not just the work they were doing, but also the difficulties that they'd had in Europe because of Greenpeace and the anti-GMO people who really made it very difficult for them to do their work. It was clear from just listening to all of this that politicians and the anti-GMO folks really needed to be educated in some way and to hear from some people — not all the false material that the Green parties were putting out, Greenpeace in particular — but to really hear about the science from some people they might listen to. So, I thought maybe the Nobel Laureates could do something there.

The day after this meeting, I was invited to go and talk to the European Commission in Brussels. I was scheduled to talk to them about the future of healthcare.

I decided that I would take the opportunity to talk to them about GMOs and the future of food. I would make the case that food was medicine. If you are hungry, food is medicine.

[57] https://theness.com/neurologicablog/index.php/farming-ideology-trumps-evidence/

[58] https://www.growmorefoundation.org/qa-with-dr-roberts

I gave a talk about GMOs that was based on that premise, and I got a very good reaction to it. An Italian senator came up to me after and said that she'd changed her mind completely on the GMO issue. She'd been anti-GMO before she heard my talk, and now she was totally pro-GMO, and really would try to do something about it. A lot of the staff members of the people that came and talked to me said that was a conversation that was not going on in Europe, and they found it very refreshing that someone like myself was talking about this.

After that, I slowly accumulated a list of Laureates who felt the way I did. At the moment, we have 129 Nobel laureates all signed onto this campaign urging Greenpeace to follow the science and stop spreading false information. Just be honest and admit this was an issue they got wrong. They do a lot of good stuff. This is one of the things they've done very badly.

You don't have to be a prize-winning scientist. Take inspiration from Julie Mellor-Trupp who went from a "GMO-hater" to biotechnology advocate. Her application of skeptical thinking was exemplary.[59] A young mother who was naturally concerned about the health of her family, she was swept up in Facebook groups which preached about the "evil Monsanto" and had her terrified of GMOs. She decided to go all-in:

> I started asking a lot of questions on my favorite forums, seeking evidence for claims that, days before, I had merely ingested as facts.
>
> I soon found out any challenge to a claim on anti-GMO sites had me being called a shill for Monsanto and permanently removed. I realized that by stifling all challenges and silencing dissent, group members forced others to fall in line, mindlessly and unquestioning. I was shocked that my months as a 'good member' meant nothing to people who now turned against me, merely for asking for evidence of their claims.

Asking questions is healthy. Doubt is healthy. Don't trust anybody who rejects your doubt, especially if they call you a shill. The idea that large

---

[59] https://geneticliteracyproject.org/2018/03/09/from-gmo-hater-to-biotechnology-advocate-one-persons-facebook-journey/

corporations spread money around on social media to get people to say nice things about them is beyond risible. (And if you have evidence that it's real, please tell me where to sign up, because they must owe me a fortune by now.)

Fear not. All food is healthy.

Chapter 3

Mythelany

Mythelany

It's time to address a potpourri of food myths. The kitchen is the heart of the home and so, not surprisingly, has accumulated a lot of folklore. There is not only fear at work, but sometimes simple ignorance or misunderstanding. Part of having a healthy relationship with food is knowing how to prepare and cook it. So let's roll up our sleeves, tie on an apron, and go all Snopes on it.

This chapter is largely an updated version of an episode[1] I did for Skeptoid,[2] a podcast which is a reliable, easy-to-digest source of information about applying science and skeptical thinking to pop culture. It's worth a subscription in your feed.

One of the things that distinguishes us from other species is our ability to cook food. I'm aware that some birds have been known to set fires by distributing burning branches,[3] but that seems to be more about frightening and driving prey than actual cooking. Our ancestors were cooking food over fires at least a million years ago, while we humans have only been around for about 300,000 years. The evolutionary advantages are huge: While most of our simian cousins have to spend a large part of their day just chewing, cooking is a form of pre-digestion that makes far

---

[1] https://skeptoid.com/episodes/4453

[2] https://skeptoid.com/

[3] https://www.sciencealert.com/birds-intentionally-set-prey-ablaze-rewriting-history-fire-use-firehawk-raptors

more nutrients, especially calories, available. That allowed our ancestors to grow these big, expensive brains. Thanks, ancestors!

So let's use our big, expensive brains to scan a list of cooking myths and see what holds up. This takes the form of pop quiz questions organized by theme. Can you guess which statements are true and which aren't?

Equipment and Technique

Grilled food is toxic — **MYTH**

This myth seems to stem from the discovery of the presence of Acrylamide in some burned foods. Later it was found to be naturally occurring in many foods. While it has been linked to toxic effects on the nervous system and fertility, the FDA and the World Health Organization found that intake would have to be some 500 times that found in an average diet to impact the nervous system, and 2,000 times to affect fertility. Remember: The dose is the poison.

Cooking in aluminum pots and pans causes Alzheimer's — **MYTH**

No link has been found between aluminum cookware and Alzheimer's. It does appear that Alzheimer's sufferers have higher concentrations of aluminum in their brains, but if aluminum exposure were the cause then Alzheimer's would be more prevalent in people with very high exposure to aluminum. And it isn't. Besides, your cookware is not a major source of aluminum intake compared to other common sources.[4] Aluminum is one of the most common elements on Earth. It's all over the place.

You should use non-reactive bowls and pans for acidic foods like sourdough and tomato sauce — **TRUE**

Cooking or preparing acidic foods in aluminum, copper, cast iron, or other reactive metals can both damage the cookware and impart a metal-

---

[4]http://www.straightdope.com/columns/read/195/does-exposure-to-aluminum-cause-alzheimers-disease/

lic taste or odd color[5] to your food. Prepare acidic foods in plastic or glass bowls, and cook in either stainless steel or non-stick pans instead.

Plastic cutting boards have fewer germs than wooden ones — **TRUE**

It turns out that a noted study claiming wood has fairly decent antibacterial properties was flawed, failing to account for bacteria hiding inside the wood and away from the surface. Wooden boards are not allowed in commercial kitchens. But are they safe for home? Well, they can be. Kept clean and well maintained,[6] either wood or plastic is a perfectly good food prep surface. The most important safety tip is to avoid cross contamination. Use separate boards for raw meats and vegetables. The USDA has a helpful web page called *Cutting Boards and Food Safety.*[7]

Whip cream and egg whites in a copper bowl if you have one, never in a plastic one — **TRUE**

Besides good heat conductivity to keep its contents cold, trace copper ions give a more stable foam. But oil molecules on the surface of plastic interfere with foam development. Glass and steel work just fine if you don't have copper. If you insist on whipping in a plastic bowl, get used to disappointment.

The microwave oven was invented when a Magnetron melted candy in a guy's pocket — **TRUE**

One day radar engineer Percy Spencer[8] noticed that the candy bar in his pocket had melted when he stood in front of an active radar. He wasn't the first to notice the effect, but he was the first to try the next logical step: Popcorn. He later enclosed the magnetron in a metal box to contain

[5] https://www.thekitchn.com/whats-the-deal-with-reactive-a-108699
[6] https://www.thespruceeats.com/cutting-boards-and-food-safety-995484
[7] https://www.fsis.usda.gov/wps/portal/fsis/topics/food-safety-education/get-answers/food-safety-fact-sheets/safe-food-handling/cutting-boards-and-food-safety
[8] https://en.wikipedia.org/wiki/Percy_Spencer

the radiation, and the microwave oven was born. Now you know why it was called the Radarange. Part of why I tell this story is to note that Spencer *was not harmed* by the microwave radiation.

Microwave ovens destroy nutrients — **MYTH**

It's easy to scare people with the word radiation. It conjures up atomic fallout, DNA damage, and random superpowers. (The latter, sadly, is also a myth. Even when delivered via spider bite.) But that damaging kind of radiation is properly called *ionizing* radiation. That's radiation with enough energy to knock electrons off of atoms or molecules, ionizing them. Ionizing radiation is made up of energetic subatomic particles, atoms moving *really* fast (like over 1% of the speed of light), or even other ions. But the electromagnetic radiation reaching your eyes right now in the form of light, and the radio waves passing through you right now, are *non-ionizing* radiation. It can't alter any molecules other than just making them wiggle faster. A molecule with a lot of wiggle is merely hotter than a quieter molecule.

The only thing the non-ionizing radiation of a microwave oven can possibly do to food is make it hotter. That's why Percy Spencer was fine: his body's natural temperature control took care of the slight warmth, but the chocolate bar warmed up just enough to get gooey. In fact, microwave heating is so gentle that it's one of the best methods, along with steaming, for *preserving* nutrients while cooking things like vegetables.

You should never heat baby formula in a microwave oven — **TRUE**

It's not because it damages the nutrients. Microwaves heat unevenly, along the microwave beam coming from the emitter (called a magnetron) and since there's no mixing from convection sometimes part of the liquid gets very hot while the surrounding liquid is cooler. So the real risk to baby is getting scalded. Shaking the bottle isn't reliably enough agitation to guarantee against it, either. So stick to a gentle stovetop method for baby's formula, and save the microwave oven for things like veggies, popcorn, and leftovers.

Alcohol completely evaporates from food when you cook it. — **MYTH**

Ethanol does boil at a lower temperature than water, but also binds with other compounds. Depending on the recipe and technique, as much as 85% of the alcohol can remain. Only very long cook times, upwards of 3 hours, are likely to remove it all. So, yes, most of the alcohol from that bottle of wine that went in the pot roast that's been in the oven for hours is probably gone, but maybe not all of it. If the recipe starts with small amounts of alcohol then this is nothing to worry about.

Salt is just salt — **MIXED**

Let's talk about salt in two contexts: cooking, and nutrition. Sure, chemically it's just Sodium Chloride. But the grain size between table salt and Kosher salt is so different that if a recipe calls specifically for one, you really don't want to substitute. A teaspoon of table salt is a lot saltier than a teaspoon of Kosher because it weighs more. Depending on the dish, the texture of the larger Kosher crystals might make a taste difference. Once dissolved in a dish, though, salt is just salt.

Some people like sea salt. That's because it has impurities which subtly alter the flavor. Don't worry, they're safe. Not quite as safe are the impurities that make Himalayan Pink Salt[9] that lovely color.[10] It gets promoted as having all sorts of magical properties, but it's really just salt with a lot of other minerals in it. I wouldn't recommend using it in cooking. And buy a pink salt lamp if you like how it looks, but it's just a lamp. Made of salt. With lots of mineral impurities.

Nutritionally we're told to minimize the sodium (principally from salt) in our diets. But getting too little salt could be worse than getting extra. Not that Americans are likely to get too little. On average they get almost three times the recommended amount of salt. Most of that comes from pre-made (so-called "processed") foods, and restaurants. Even breakfast cereals can carry quite a bit of it. The good news is that if you cook at home you can pretty much add as much salt as you

[9] https://sciencebasedmedicine.org/pass-the-salt-but-not-that-pink-himalayan-stuff/
[10] https://sciencebasedmedicine.org/pink-himalayan-sea-salt-an-update/

want because you'll end up with far less than what's hiding in packaged foods. Those foods often use salt as a preservative, so if you eat a lot of them you get used to a saltier taste. Home cooking won't have that problem.

Do not listen to anybody trying to frighten you away from salt. It isn't a toxin trying to kill you. You just need to moderate your intake.

Does going easy on salt pay off? The answer is a qualified yes. As Dr. Novella points out:[11]

> [T]he current consensus is something like this:
> - Most of the world, including Americans and those in industrialized nations, consume more salt than appears to be necessary.
> - In the US most of that salt comes from processed or restaurant food (while in other countries, like Japan, most salt intake is added while cooking).
> - There is a plausible connection between excess salt intake, hypertension, strokes and heart attacks.
> - There is evidence to suggest that reducing overall salt intake will reduce the incidence of these health problems, but the evidence is not yet conclusive and longer term and subpopulation data is needed.

Vinegar never goes bad — **TRUE**

Good news for your food budget, right? *Cook's Illustrated* magazine tested 12-year-old balsamic. It was fine. Old vinegar may have a harmless sediment lurking in the bottom of the bottle. Stir it up, filter it out, or just ignore it. Don't throw away old vinegar. This is also a fine excuse to keep a variety of vinegars around. Note that vinegar is just vinegar. None of it is magical, and you shouldn't drink it straight. Some outrageous claims are made for apple cider vinegar. Ignore those. It's just vinegar. But tasty!

---

[11] https://sciencebasedmedicine.org/the-war-on-salt/

Limes have lots of Vitamin C — **MIXED**

Like all citrus, they have some. But only half as much as lemons. You shouldn't really be choosing your produce based on vitamin content anyway. Just eat a variety, enjoy it, and you'll get all the Vitamin C you need.

Cooking vegetables robs them of nutrition — **MYTH**

The "raw is better" idea is really another facet of the naturalistic fallacy. Enthusiasts will point out that raw vegetables have all their enzymes intact. While this is true, the acids in your stomach will thoroughly destroy any that weren't rinsed away when you washed them. (You do wash your vegetables, I hope.) Besides, the plants need the enzymes to grow, but they're of no particular use to you. On the contrary, cooking food is why humans extract nutrients from our food more efficiently than our poor simian cousins, some of whom have to spend a third of their day chewing.

Don't let that discourage you from enjoying vegetables and fruits that can be eaten raw, of course. Many are delicious that way.

Brightly colored vegetables are the most nutritious — **MYTH**

I kind of wanted this one to be true. To me a bright, colorful salad is a thing of beauty. Well, it still is. After all, we eat first with our eyes. But how brightly colored a vegetable is has no correlation with how many or what kind of nutrients are aboard. Many pale veggies (especially beans) are packed with all kinds of goodness. Remember, too, that since there is no single-axis metric for "nutritious" it's impossible to call one food more nutritious than another anyway.

Bread goes stale because it dries out — **MYTH**

Surprising, right? Actually it's just the opposite. One of the things I love about bread, besides the joy of eating it, is that it represents some truly fascinating chemistry. The bread is absorbing moisture, actually getting heavier. The moisture causes the starch granules to crystalize, hardening the bread. That's why you don't keep bread in the refrigerator, and why a brief visit to the oven can soften it again. Staling is quite a different process than drying out, which is why you can't rescue stale bread by dunking it in water.

Beans make you fart — **TRUE**

Indeed beans, and a long list of other foods high in fiber and/or polysaccharides, can contribute to flatulence. This can be mitigated with a few techniques. The Exploratorium lists some good ones:[12]

- A most sensible tactic involves a lengthy soaking, and was developed some years ago by the California Dry Bean Advisory Board. For each pound of dried beans, use ten or more cups of boiling water. Boil for two to three minutes, cover, and set the beans aside overnight. This initial boiling breaks down the cell membranes of the beans, releasing the oligosaccharides so they can dissolve into the soaking water. Just make sure you discard the soaking water!

- Cook beans well before adding any acidic ingredients like tomatoes or molasses, as acids prevent legumes from softening. When beans are softer, they're also more digestible.

- Try an over-the-counter digestive aid, such as Beano, which contains the sugar-digesting enzyme that the body lacks. Use Beano just before eating so it can break down the gas-producing oligosaccharides. It has no effect, however, on gas caused by lactose or fiber.

- Try adding epazote (1 tablespoon to a large pot of chili, beans, or soup). Epazote is the leaf of a wild herb, prized for its gas-reducing abilities. [I'll add that epazote is also very tasty, and if you try it you might just discover that it's a "secret ingredient" to some of your favorite Mexican food.]

Pasta has collected a number of myths. Here are a few:

[12] http://www.exploratorium.edu/cooking/icooks/4-1-03-article.html

*You should add salt to the water to make it boil faster. — **FALSE***

While it's true that water with salt in it boils at a lower temperature than plain water, the difference it makes is so tiny that you need lab equipment to find it. You shouldn't be using all that much salt in the first place. But do salt the water some: it helps the flavor.

*Put a lid on the pot to make it boil faster — **MIXED***

This makes a tiny bit of difference, but only after the water is close to the boiling point. On those hungry-now-gimme-my-pasta nights feel free to start heating the pot of water and then look for the lid.

*Adding olive oil keeps the pasta from sticking, or the water from boiling over — **MYTHS***

Oil and water don't mix. It won't prevent boiling over, but will give you slimy pasta that sauce doesn't want to stick to. And it's a waste of olive oil.

*You should never rinse your pasta — **TRUE***

You want that starchy water to act as an emulsifier to help your sauce adhere to the pasta. Many recipes, and all pasta restaurants, actually reserve some of that water for saucing. If it's cloudy with starch that's the good stuff.

*You need a large pot of boiling water to cook pasta — **MYTH***

This is one that I believed for a long time. Surprisingly, you not only don't need much water, but it doesn't even have to be boiling the whole time! Chef J. Kenji López-Alt developed a wonderful technique for cooking dry pasta, which he describes on The Food Lab.[13] You should read it, but here's the tl;dr — Bring a small amount of salted water to a boil, stir in

---

[13] https://www.seriouseats.com/2010/05/how-to-cook-pasta-salt-water-boiling-tips-the-food-lab.html

the dry pasta, cover, and then turn off the heat. Yes, off! In the normal cooking time you'll not only have terrific pasta, but really starchy water for saucing. Experiment with it and you'll be surprised at how little water you need. Note that you're also saving both energy and time, because a small pot of water boils a lot sooner than a big one, lid or no lid.

And now, on to some dairy and seafood myths:

European eggs don't need refrigeration — **TRUE**

But their eggs are sold unwashed, and Europeans tend to buy in small quantities and consume their eggs quickly. Properly refrigerated, eggs have a really good shelf life anyway.

Cheese never goes bad - you can just cut off the mold — **MIXED**

Hard cheeses are usually fine for quite a while under the mold. Soft cheeses, like bleu cheese, not so much. Cheese stores best cool and dry, not sealed in a bag where it can collect moisture.

Raw milk is healthier than pasteurized. — **MYTH**

What it really is, is risky. Their are no significant nutritional advantages to raw milk, and the serious health risks aren't worth the small flavor advantage. Raw milk enthusiasts typically represent another facet of the naturalistic, "raw is better" fallacy. They can get downright religious in their fervor. They can also get Brucella, Listeria, Mycobacterium bovis (a cause of tuberculosis), Salmonella, Shigella, Yersinia, Giardia, and norovirus.[14] Worse, so can their kids.

A recent review article[15] has shown that much of what we think we know about milk is wrong. Like that there's no correlation between milk consumption and body weight. Its relationship to diabetes is uncertain, with some studies showing that it *lowers* risk. And how's this for a surprising conclusion:

---

[14] https://sciencebasedmedicine.org/raw-milk-in-modern-times/
[15] https://sciencebasedmedicine.org/milk-and-health-the-evidence/

"Milk doesn't "build strong bones" but may actually increase the risk of fracture. There's no evidence that reduced-fat milk has any health advantages over whole milk.

Never wash your chicken — **TRUE**

Poultry (or, as I like to think of it, *edible dinosaurs*) is the only meat commonly processed with the skin on. That's why it can harbor dangerous microbes such as salmonella. If you wash it, you aren't disinfecting it at all, but spreading germs all over the sink, your hands, and the kitchen. Cooking it is the best way to pasteurize it. Make sure it all hits a safe temperature.

Lobsters scream when you boil them — **MYTH**

That sound is steam rapidly escaping their shells. The separate question, do they feel pain, is still unsettled. Many think that such a simple nervous system is incapable of it. While some scientists find that they do feel pain, other scientists question the validity[16] of their methods. The answer for now seems to be that we just don't know.

Fish comes from an environment about the same temperature as your refrigerator, which is why it spoils faster than meat — **TRUE**

Keeping fish properly chilled is important for both safety and flavor. That's why good fish shops pack it in ice for you. If you want to enjoy any raw fish, you need to treat temperature and freshness as critical items, and also put a *lot* of faith in your fishmonger. Even something that says "sushi grade" on it might not be, if it hasn't been handled properly.

Finally, the food that has to be the source of the most common and persistent myths: Meat.

---

[16]http://www.straightdope.com/columns/read/2837/do-lobsters-feel-pain-when-boiled-alive

*Pork needs to be cooked well-done — **MYTH***

The risk of trichinosis, a parasitic disease, has all but vanished in the
United States and many other parts of the world. The USDA has even re-
vised the minimum safe temperature[17] for pork downward to 145° F (63°
C). This is great news because pork is a fairly lean meat, and overcooking
just makes it tough and dry.

*Leftover meat needs to be reheated — **MIXED***

It's safe to eat cold leftovers if they were rapidly cooled after cooking.
Bacteria in the presence of air can reproduce in a temperature range
between 40° F and 140° F (5° C - 60°C). If it stayed out on the counter
for a couple of hours[18] before hitting the fridge, consider a thorough
reheat[19].

*Red juice leaking from a burger means it's not safe — **MYTH***

No, that's not blood, and no, it doesn't mean the burger is undercooked.
The doneness of meat is entirely a function of temperature. Beef that
isn't overcooked should still have plenty of juices. It's true that ground
meat is safer cooked all the way to medium, or 140° F (60° C) than at
medium rare. Steaks are safe at medium rare (132° F, 55°C) because the
interior hasn't been exposed to the air. Once beef passes medium, it's
really not getting any safer or any better cooked. The proteins are just
contracting, getting tougher, and squeezing out the juices — along with
a lot of the flavor.

*You can test the doneness of steak by pressing it with a finger — **MYTH***

OK, all of you restaurant kitchen denizens, just calm down. Many professional cooks claim to be able to do this, and they do probably get away

---

[17] http://www.webmd.com/food-recipes/news/20110525/cooking-temperatures-for-pork
[18] https://www.theskepticsguide.org/ask-the-skeptic-reheating-meat
[19] https://www.foodsafety.gov/keep-food-safe/4-steps-to-food-safety#cook

with it. They have the advantage not only of experience, but familiarity with the cut of beef and their cooking equipment. An accurate, instant-read thermometer inserted into it is the only way to *accurately* know how done a piece of meat is. It's kitchen hardware that I highly recommend. It will make you a better cook.

Don't turn a steak with a fork, or cut it open to check it, or the juices will run out — **MYTH**

But you can see juices coming out, right? Yes, but not enough to make a difference. This is trivially proven by weighing the steaks before and after. That's exactly what *Cook's Illustrated* did when they busted this myth. Steaks aren't bags and they don't spring leaks.

Drum roll, please! This has to be the most stubborn myth in the kitchenverse, the king of all everybody-knows cooking falsehoods:

Searing meat seals in the juices — **MYTH**

Quite the opposite is the case. Heating meat always causes proteins to contract, which always squeezes out some juices. What that quick sear does is provoke the Maillard reaction. This is the same chemical change that happens when you toast bread or brown food in general. Amino acids and sugars react to form hundreds (seriously — *hundreds*) of flavor compounds, giving just about anything a real flavor boost. As you learn to cook you'll doubtless hear more about the Maillard reaction. It's one of your best friends in the kitchen!

I don't know about you, but this chapter made me kind of hungry. If you want to take a break, head into the kitchen, and whip up something yummy, please be my guest.

Chapter 4

Choosing What to Eat

Nutrition 101

As I mentioned earlier, foods are different, get processed differently by our bodies, and in different ways and at different speeds. The science of nutrition is amazingly complex and hard to study in detail. Fortunately, though, there's a perfectly useful and simple way to look at it which is all we, the eaters of the world, need to know in order to make healthy food choices. We'll leave the technical details to the scientists who continue to push the edges of our understanding. The basic consensus has been quite consistent for decades now. That's why I'm comfortable suggesting that you just enjoy a variety of foods, mostly plants, including plenty of vegetables and fruits, not too much or too little.

Let's look at what all foods have in common, and then look at the differences that matter to us.

The same seven things.

No matter how varied our diet, no matter how complex the chemistry and interactions, everything you eat basically just gives you some combination of these seven basic things:

1. Carbohydrates
2. Proteins
3. Fats
4. Hydration
5. Vitamins

6. Minerals
7. Fiber

Looked at this way it's clear why no foods have magical "health benefits" and why there are no superfoods. There are just foods. Let's get an overview of the Big Seven and see how it applies to how we choose what to eat, and when.

The first three are known as the *macro nutrients*. Besides hydration (a fancy word for what water gives you) the most vital nutrition your body needs is something that provides calories. Never forget that calories are good, not evil. Without enough calories you sicken and die a horribly painful death. The trick, as we've already discussed, is not maintaining a long term calorie surplus, because eventually that will cause enough weight gain to put you at risk for several poor health outcomes.

Carbohydrates are molecules that consist of just Carbon, Oxygen, and Hydrogen. There are usually twice as many Hydrogens as Oxygens — the same ratio as in water. Carbs are really good at storing energy and releasing it quickly. That's why plants use energy from sunlight to combine CO_2 (Carbon Dioxide) and H_2O (water) to make carbohydrates. And that's why we eat plants, harvest the energy stored in those carbs, and release CO_2 and water. Yes, you really are solar powered. Congratulations.

The smallest carbs, as in the ones with the smallest molecular weight, are usually called sugars. Maybe you think of sugar as just one thing and, in terms of how you eat, that's usually adequate. Sugars are such awesome energy delivery molecules that your body pretty much runs on them. Your brain, especially, runs preferentially on glucose.

We don't have to delve deep into the chemistry of monosaccharides vs. disaccharides. It's enough for now to know that the simpler ones, such as fructose and glucose are monosaccharides and sucrose (which is the sugar you buy in granulated form at the store) is a disaccharide. Organic chemistry is wicked complicated and science has a lot of naming conventions. Let's keep it simple and note that most chemical names ending in *-ose* are sugars. So when you're reading a label and see *dextrose*, you can just think "some kind of sugar". Simple, no? (Dextrose happens to be another name for glucose. Go figure.)

The other thing to note about the mono- and di- forms of sugar is that your body will turn the di- (sucrose) into its component sugars, namely fructose and glucose. And now you know why "high fructose corn syrup" (HFCS) is really just another name for "sugar", because it turns into fructose and glucose in your body just like regular sugar does, except with a slightly higher proportion of fructose.

Fructose, you've doubtless guessed from the name, is the sugar we primarily find in fruit. There's nothing wrong with fructose. Different sugars have different perceived sweetness, and fructose tastes sweeter than glucose or sucrose, meaning you could theoretically use less sugar if you sweeten your food with HFCS. I mention this because a lot of people are going to try to convince you that HFCS in your food will curse you and your children, make you hate puppies, and give you cancer. Or something else bad.

Nah. It's just sugar.

Complex carbohydrates are just bigger molecules that can break down into sugars. Carbs are, as I said, great energy sources. Your body can turn them into useful energy very quickly. The simpler the carb, the faster the body can glom onto those calories. Say you're a bicycle racer. (Go on. Say "you're a bicycle racer". Let the person next to you wonder what the book you're reading is about. It could be a great conversation starter.) You're about to pedal like mad for a hundred miles or so. Many such athletes will sit down to a gargantuan serving of pasta before the race, a process known as carb loading. In short order that fuel is converted to the sugars that power muscles. You've probably heard the claim that pasta is fattening, so why don't bicycle racers waddle around, spandex stretched to the point of destruction? Because pasta *isn't* fattening, of course. No food is. Also because they output so much energy that they burn it all off before it can be stored. An olympic swimmer can easily put away over 10,000 calories per day, and they aren't exactly tubby, either.

Those of us who aren't olympic athletes need to moderate our sugar and even carbohydrate input. That's largely to stay in calorie balance, but there are other concerns. Sugars, especially, can form a surplus very quickly. You thought your liver was busy clearing toxins and waste products, and it is, but it also gets the job of quick sugar storage. It makes fat that can also be broken down relatively quickly into sugars for the body, but if your diet overdoes the sugars it can get overwhelmed to the point that your doctor may tell you to whoa up on the soda because you have a "fatty liver".

Large spikes in sugar also tax your body's insulin system. That's a hormone that regulates the absorption of carbohydrates, fats, and proteins (all your macros). If you down a lot of sweets at once you get a quick sugar spike. If it's infrequent, or if you're very active at the time, this is not a big deal. Cumulatively, though, you can give your pancreas (in charge of insulin) and liver a hard time. I don't know about you, but I'd rather have a mellow, happy pancreas and liver.

As we already covered in the *Sugar isn't Cocaine and Bacon Won't Give You Cancer* section of the **All Food is Healthy** chapter, this is why you should keep your daily average below 5% of your TDEE or, round numbers for most adults, around 25 grams of added sugar. It's also why you shouldn't have soda or fruit juice too frequently. Nutritionally they're pretty much the same thing: water and sugar. Juice may also have some vitamins. So while it's fine to juice your fruits and veggies now and then, go easy on it. Even blending food into a smoothie (and who doesn't love a good smoothie?) makes the sugars much more instantly available. So go for it, just maybe not every day.

So why don't we worry about all that sugar in fruits? I mean, here I've been telling you to eat lots of fruit and then I tell you they're full of sugar. What's up with that? Here's what.

Fruits don't really have a large dose of sugar in them. That's why even a big, juicy, sweet summer peach isn't even 100 calories, and why an orange may have only around 60 or 70 calories. But that 8-ounce glass of orange juice? That has the juice, and the calories, of between 2 and 4 oranges. Compare those 110 calories to the 97 calories in 8 ounces of Coca-Cola and you can begin to see my point. Would I personally rather have orange juice? Most of the time, you betcha. But I'm going to watch how much I have, and how frequently. And if you want a Coke now and then, by all means go ahead. It's just sugar.

Whole fruits have a lot of fiber. We'll talk more about what fiber does for us later. For now one cool trick it does in fruit is called *buffering*. What that means is that it greatly slows down how quickly the fructose can get absorbed into your system. It's why you don't have to worry about sugar spikes while munching fruit.

So carbohydrates are just a normal, natural food macro. When you know that you need a lot of energy right away for a high level of physical activity, consider complex carbs your BFF. There's nothing wrong with carbs, and there is no reason to eliminate them from your diet. Beware anybody saying that you should. Just don't overdo it.

Proteins are a varied range of complex molecules made up of animo acids. They're the basic building blocks of our bodies, to oversimplify for a book about food and drive biochemist readers to distraction. For our purposes there are only a few key things you need to know about proteins. One is that you need them in your diet. Your body can do different things with proteins that you eat. One is it breaks them down into amino acids that it can use to build the proteins it wants. An obvious example is building muscle. It can also break proteins down even further and turn them into fuel. As a fuel, protein has about the same calorie density as carbohydrates.

Proteins are considered an essential nutrient because there are nine amino acids that the body needs and can't make on its own. Their names are phenylalanine, valine, threonine, tryptophan, methionine, leucine, isoleucine, lysine, and histidine. (I can't decide if those should be super-hero names or a wicked cool law firm.) There are six more known as con-ditionally essential amino acids because people with certain conditions can't make enough of their own: arginine, cysteine, glycine, glutamine, proline and tyrosine. We're not going much deeper into the chemistry rab-bit hole, but if your curiosity is piqued you can look them up on Wikipedia. For our purposes, we just know that if we don't get enough of those amino acids (from protein in our diet) we run the risk of malnutrition.

A famously vegan friend of mine complains that the first question he gets about his diet from people is "where do you get your protein?".

Getting enough protein isn't hard. If you eat a varied diet you'll get plenty. Everybody knows that animal products such as fish, eggs, meat and dairy are rich in proteins, but protein abounds in plant life as well. You get protein from grains, legumes, nuts, and seeds — all of which should be part of your varied diet as long as you have no allergies. There are those who preach a "carbs bad, protein good" kind of religion but, as we know, there is no bad food, and most people get plenty of protein. It's usually not a worry, and there's no need to supplement your diet with protein powder or protein shakes unless, maybe, you're a body builder bulking up.

Unlike carbs, which the body can digest and absorb lickety-split, proteins take a while to process. That's a big part of why they provide more satiety (the nutritionist's word for "stickin' to yer ribs") than carbs. More satiety means it takes longer for you to feel hungry. This can be useful in different contexts.

One is just plain not overeating. If your meals include a decent amount of protein you're more likely to feel satisfied for longer, and may end up skipping those snacks that are pushing the envelope on your calorie budget.

Another is getting better sleep. If you go to bed hungry, your brain's hunger cues can arouse you enough to interrupt your sleep quality but not enough to rouse you out of bed to raid the fridge. A doctor helping you with insomnia, or one treating you for an eating disorder (which can also wreak havoc on sleep) may suggest an evening snack rich in proteins and fats (which also digest slowly) just to keep your brain from getting the noms while you're in dreamland.

So our friends the proteins are essential for our health, keep us from feeling hungry, and are trivial to get in a varied diet. They are not magical, and it's rather unlikely that you have to worry about not getting enough of them.

Fats get a bad rap. Remember that old saw, "you are what you eat"? Well, you aren't. And fat doesn't make you fat. It's a nutrient that has the highest calorie density of any food so, obviously, a diet with a *lot* of fat might be a fattening one. It's actually a good thing to get a variety of fats in your diet but, to an even greater degree than proteins, you don't have to go hunting for it. Most Americans are getting more than they need.

I'm never going to give you a list of foods that you shouldn't eat, and recommend that you cast a jaundiced eye at anybody who does. There are, though, some ingredients you'll want to minimize as part of your daily diet. A couple of them are certain types of fat. Let's take a look and try not to get distracted by the chemistry.

Trans fats[1] are a kind of unsaturated fat that occurs relatively infre-

---

[1] https://en.wikipedia.org/wiki/Trans_fat

quently in nature but which was concentrated in some industrialized foods such as vegetable shortening and margarine. Getting small, or infrequent, amounts is not a problem. When the link between overconsumption of trans fats and coronary artery disease became the scientific consensus the WHO recommended that it be reduced to trace amounts, no more than 1% of your diet. World wide there's an effort to completely remove them from the food supply. Current FDA regulations severely restrict the use of trans fats in foods so avoiding them in the U.S. isn't much of a challenge now.

Saturated fats[2] are typically found in animal products, though they also occur in some vegetables. The current science on its health impact is somewhat mixed, but leaning toward a low saturated fat diet. If you get enough variety and don't skip the veggies then it's highly improbable that you'll get an unhealthy dose. Foods high in saturated fats include pizza, sausage, and ice cream. Make those special occasion foods and not staples. This isn't rocket science.

Cholesterol: You were wondering why I haven't mentioned cholesterol yet, right? Aren't there supposed to be "good cholesterol" and "bad cholesterol"? And those are fats, right? The reason is that, while there's a relatively good scientific consensus that cholesterol is a contributing factor in arterial sclerosis, the whole question of what cholesterol you *eat* is still quite up in the air. It's not true that the cholesterol in your food goes straight into your blood stream. Just like it does with proteins, your body breaks down lipids (what scientists call fats) and builds the ones it wants. So the cholesterol you eat is not the cholesterol you get. For that reason the best suggestion now is to not even think about cholesterol and just limit the proportion of fat in your diet.

There are people out there telling you to get zero fat in your diet, that all oils are bad for you. There are others shouting that fats are great and that sugar is the real problem. By this point in the book I imagine you can see the problem with both of those positions. Any time someone tries to blame (or credit) one food or ingredient for a whole host of conditions you can give them a smug *akshully* about over-simplification. And if you scratch their web site, dollars to doughnuts you'll find a shopping cart.

---

[2] https://en.wikipedia.org/wiki/Saturated_fat

Real nutrition science is messier than that. Dr. Steven Novella gives a good summary:[3]

> There isn't as much discussion about cholesterol anymore. The debate now focuses on fat in the diet. It's clear that the old recommendation of an overall low-fat diet [was] too simplistic. There are different kinds of fat, as I mentioned above. LDL transports fat from the liver to the blood vessel walls, while HDL transports fat from the blood vessels to the liver. Therefore, LDL bad, and HDL good.
>
> So the question became – which kinds of dietary fats increase LDL and/or lower HDL? The current consensus, represented by the AHA [American Heart Association], is that saturated fats, trans-fats, and hydrogenated fats all increase LDL. Polyunsaturated fats increase HDL. Monounsaturated fats may increase HDL a bit, but not as much as polyunsaturated, and perhaps not enough to have a health impact.
>
> There is ongoing debate about the relative impact of LDL vs HDL and their ratio. Coconut oil, for example, is high in saturated fat, and increases both LDL and HDL. The AHA recommendation to avoid coconut oil comes from evidence that raising LDL has more of an impact [on] vascular risk than raising HDL.
>
> There is not that much controversy over the relationship between saturated and polyunsaturated fats and LDL/HDL profiles. The real controversy is over the impact this has on vascular risk, and that was the focus of much of the backlash against the AHA report. Critics argue that the evidence for a net health benefit (longer survival, for example) from lowering dietary saturated fat is slim.

Like I said, the science is messy. One trap you shouldn't fall for after reading this book is what I call the Fat of the Month Club. Recently it was coconut oil. Sometimes it's olive oil (extra virgin, of course) or fish oil. Remember that it's not true that if a little is good more is better. That's why I stress variety and proportion.

---

[3] https://sciencebasedmedicine.org/the-skinny-on-saturated-fat/

The bottom line on fat is, then: avoid trans fats, keep saturated fats low, and keep your variety up. Remember that what you eat today doesn't matter. Never feel guilty about food, and certainly don't beat yourself up about enjoying a celebration now and then. Have whatever you want on Thanksgiving. Just make sure your regular diet has a healthy variety and proportion and you'll be fine.

Hydration is your most critical nutrition. Most people can survive weeks or more with no food. Being without water can kill you in days. Conversely, getting too much water all at once will also kill you. Don't worry — you have to do something stupid like down a gallon or more all at once for it to result in water toxicity.

One of the most persistent food myths is the old saw that you should drink 8 glasses of water per day. Well, not so fast. It really depends mostly on the climate and your level of physical activity. The 8 glasses myth apparently started with a 1945 recommendation from the Food and Nutrition Board of the National Research Council. They indeed said that an average adult needs about 8 glasses of water per day. The part that gets left out is that they also said, "Most of this quantity is contained in prepared foods." That's right: most of the food you eat contains water. Some fruits and vegetables are almost *all* water. So, no, you don't need to stand at the sink downing 8 glasses of water every day. Doing it all at once wouldn't do much more than stress your kidneys anyway.

So how much water should you drink? Gosh. If only there were a reliable way to know.

Wait. There is.

Drink when you're thirsty.

That's about it. And no, being thirsty doesn't mean you're already dehydrated. That's another myth. It just means that your body could use some water. (An early symptom of actual dehydration is often a headache.) Please don't use this advice to minimize your water intake. If you feel like having some water or another beverage, have it. Staying well hydrated is a healthy habit, and lowers your risk of things like kidney stones. You really don't want those. Ask me how I know.

You've probably heard the coffee dehydration myth, a claim that drinking coffee will actually dehydrate you because caffeine is a diuretic (fancy word for *pee inducing*). Well, technically it is a mild diuretic. But it most certainly does not take more water out of your body than the coffee put in. Ditto for any other beverage someone tries to tell you will be dehydrating. Pretty much all of them, water, milk, juice, soda, sports drinks, coffee, and tea, are primarily made of water. They all hydrate you.

The simplest way to know if you're adequately hydrated is notice when you pee. If it's multiple times in a day then you're probably fine. If you drink a full glass of a beverage and find you need to urinate an hour or so later, you're really fine.

If you live in a mild climate, eat a normal diet, and have a normal amount of activity, odds are you'll never know what dehydration feels like. Which is a good thing, because it's a lot worse than just being really thirsty. I live in central coastal California and my doctor told me I'd actually have to work at getting dehydrated here. If you're a Marine running around in the desert hauling 80 pounds of battle rattle, you're going to need way more than those 8 glasses of water. But that's really not a common case for most people. Keep eating that varied diet (fruits and veggies have lots of water in them) and drink when you're thirsty. That's about all you need to know about hydration.

Vitamins and minerals are the micro nutrients. They really are micro because, while you need many grams per day of the macro nutrients, your micro nutrient needs are in the milligrams. Vitamins are chemicals that your body needs but that it can't synthesize on its own. That's really about all they have in common. They're made by plants and animals. And minerals are, in our context, elements that the body needs and which have to come from the earth. We get them, just like vitamins, in the foods we eat and the water we drink.

The major dietary minerals for humans are calcium, phosphorus, potassium, sodium, and magnesium. The rest are known as "trace elements": sulfur, iron, chlorine, cobalt, copper, zinc, manganese, molybdenum, iodine, and selenium. Your body uses them in a variety of processes. Iron, for example, is used in hemoglobin to transport oxygen around in your blood.

As you'll find when you get to the *Beware Bad Advice* chapter, you don't need to supplement your intake of vitamins and minerals except under extraordinary circumstances. A diet with even a modicum of variety will supply you with all the micro nutrients you need.

Fiber is an odd case. By definition, in a nutritional context, it's the part of foods that you can't digest nor absorb, or at least not very well. So why do you need it? As we already talked about in our sugar discussion, it can buffer the absorption of nutrients, especially sugars. But that's a small part of the picture.

Dietary fiber can be divided roughly into two groups: soluble, or fermentable fiber, and insoluble fiber. Both play multiple roles in the amazing chemical processing plant that is your digestive tract. In fact, exactly what's going on in there and how fiber plays into it is currently a very active area of investigation. We do have a pretty good idea of a few things.

Insoluble fiber, or at least much of it, performs a bulking function which helps keep you regular, among other things. It may be that insufficient fiber contributes to an increased risk of diverticulitis (lesions that are like little pouches) but the science isn't yet clear on that.

Soluble fiber is part of the food for your gut microbiome. It, and the microorganisms it feeds, play a complex role in regulating nutrient absorption and, well, a whole lot of stuff. I'm going all vague here because the science is still pretty new.

A good summary of what, as of this writing, we know about the gut microbiome is that it varies a lot by individual, is probably very important, and is an exciting and promising field for research. Recent findings suggest that it may be more an indicator of your health than a cause of it.

You've probably already noticed that "can be optimized using the right products" is not on that list. That doesn't keep a lot of companies from trying, though. They'll try to sell you probiotics (which may or may not even survive more than a few minutes in your stomach, and which have no established role or benefits anyway) or other products designed to alter or tune your gut flora and fauna somehow. There simply is no scientific consensus yet[4] on how, or if, that can, or should, be done. Some recent studies[5] are finding that probiotics, when they aren't just uselessly pooped out, may actually be doing harm. One small study even shows

---

[4] https://www.cell.com/cell/fulltext/S0092-8674(18)31102-4
[5] https://www.cbc.ca/radio/quirks/nov-3-2018-politics-puts-the-amazon-at-risk-the-problem-with-probiotics-biggest-bird-was-blind-and-more-1.4887843/probiotics-

risks of colonizing your gut with the wrong bacteria, leading to "brain fogginess and bloating".[6]

I would not be surprised, given the amount of research going on, if in a few years we had credible advice on the care and feeding of our gut microbiome. It's pretty safe to say that effective probiotic treatments will be individualized, and not the one-size-fits-all products being hawked in stores and on line now.[7] That is if effective probiotics ever become a thing.

For now the advice is simple: Make sure there's a variety of fiber in your diet. And how do you do that? Variety, of course. Make sure that variety includes whole vegetables, fruits, and grains.

Soluble sources of fiber, in varying amounts, include:

- Legumes, such as peas, soybeans, lupins, and other beans
- Oats, rye, chia, and barley
- Many fruits, such as figs, avocados, plums, prunes, berries, ripe bananas, and the skins of apples, quinces, and pears
- Lots of vegetables such as broccoli, carrots, and Jerusalem artichokes
- Root tubers and root vegetables such as sweet potatoes and onions and their skins
- Psyllium seed husks and flax seeds
- Nuts, with almonds being the highest in dietary fiber

Insoluble fiber sources include:

- Whole grain foods
- Wheat and corn bran
- Legumes such as beans and peas
- Nuts and seeds
- Potato skins
- Vegetables such as green beans, cauliflower, zucchini, celery, and nopal

probably-aren-t-making-you-well-and-they-could-make-you-sicker-1.4887860
   [6]https://medicalxpress.com/news/2018-08-probiotic-link-brain-fogginess-severe.html
   [7]https://www.smithsonianmag.com/science-nature/benefits-probiotics-might-not-be-so-clear-cut-180970221/

- Various fruits including avocado, and unripe bananas
- The skins of some fruits, including kiwifruit, grapes, and tomatoes

Did you notice that some foods appear in both lists? That's part of why I say that if you get enough variety you're almost sure to get enough fiber. It's also a reminder not to choose foods because of a specific nutrient. In case your doctor suggests it, though, there are fiber supplements, usually flavored powders of psyllium husk, that can help with certain conditions. Taken as directed they're quite safe. Those of us of a certain age, particularly if we were less than vigilant about food in our youth, may want to supplement fiber a bit. As always, check with your medical doctor to be sure.

This is far from an exhaustive look at everything fiber is doing in your gut. Like I said at the outset, this isn't a science book. Feel free to take a deep dive starting on Wikipedia[8] if you'd like to know more. It's all fascinating, but doesn't affect how we decide what to eat.

Congratulations on completing your Nutrition 101 course. Let's take this basic knowledge and start figuring out how to eat — and what nutritional advice to ignore.

Eating for Active People

Athletes have, or at least seem to have, special dietary requirements. Obviously more output requires more fuel, so there's that. I already mentioned that some athletes do "carbo loading", eating a lot of complex carbs right before a high output activity. If it's the right activity, that's a fine thing to do, but don't do it big time unless a sports medicine doctor has recommended it.

Athletes as a group are, unfortunately, very superstitious. You should probably not get dietary advice from athletes no matter how fit. I'll throw in most coaches as well. Beware advice from companies selling "sports drinks" or "recovery drinks" as well. We won't make a deep dive into the subject, but the bottom line is that you don't need them unless you're a professional or high-performance athlete. And even then you don't need a lot of the things people push at you.

---

[8] https://en.wikipedia.org/wiki/Dietary_fiber

Sports drink companies, starting with Gatorade, have pushed the idea of hydration to a dangerous degree. Nobody has ever died of dehydration running a marathon, but several have died from over-hydration. We'll discuss what that means and how it happens in the section on Water Woo in the *Beware Bad Advice* chapter. The idea that if you're thirsty you're already dehydrated is a myth, as is the idea that you need to drink a lot of water while you work out. It turns out that your body, evolved as it is to be able to hunt in packs, running down prey, naturally retains water during a long run or workout. Have some water afterwards if you're thirsty. Likely you will be. And don't worry about replacing electrolytes (fancy word for salts) with a sports drink. The salt you get in your diet is fine.

The idea that you need protein supplements, such as Muscle Milk or protein powders, for workout recovery is a myth started by (I hope you're sitting down) someone who realized that there was more money in selling supplements for years than barbells once. In any case you can only absorb so much protein at a time, and it's better to get your protein from food, spread throughout the day.

The best recovery from exercise is a healthy diet and plenty of good sleep. Working out doesn't leave your body depleted in any special way, other than burning calories and losing a little extra water. Here again are where cravings, if you're paying careful attention, can help. If you really want something salty it could be because you need some salt. And, it bears repeating, if you're thirsty it means that you should drink something, not that you're already dehydrated.

One thing elite athletes have in common with the rest of us is that there is no scientific evidence of an optimal, ideal diet. There isn't even evidence that specific foods help performance. The best evidence that any dietary fine tuning provides very small effects is that no experiments have shown significant effects for anything. We're all omnivores, and we can all do fine on a variety of foods.

Beware the Latest Study

Being a Smart Science Consumer

Science is complicated. Medical and nutritional science are crazy complicated. Thankfully, though, science is a self-correcting method of investigation, so it gradually gets closer and closer to the right answers. This is reflected in a growing consensus. It's easy to confuse *consensus* with *voting*. No, scientists don't vote on what reality is. Reality doesn't care what anybody's opinion is. But when multiple lines of evidence and a large body of high quality research all converge in a way that the vast majority of experts in a field agree on something, that's a scientific consensus.

When evaluating science about nutrition it's really important to look for that consensus position. Not only is it the most likely to be correct, but it isn't going to change day-to-day or even likely year-to-year. You could go crazy trying to keep up with the latest studies. Not only that, you could be wrong. Remember how I said that science was self-correcting? That's perhaps its best feature, but it leads to a counter-intuitive result.

Most Scientific Studies are Wrong

This isn't necessarily a bad thing. Let's wrap our heads around what this means. In 2015 a Stanford health researcher named John Iaonnidis surveyed the landscape of scientific papers and published *Why Most Published Research Findings Are False*[9]. His abstract is pretty clear:

> There is increasing concern that most current published research findings are false. The probability that a research claim is true may depend on study power and bias, the number of other studies on the same question, and, importantly, the ratio of true to no relationships among the relationships probed in each scientific field. In this framework, a research finding is less likely to be true when the studies conducted in a field are smaller; when effect sizes are smaller; when there is a greater number and lesser preselection of tested relationships; where there is greater flexibility in designs, definitions, outcomes, and analytical modes; when there is greater financial and other interest and prejudice; and when more teams are involved in a scientific field in chase of statistical significance. Simulations show that for most study designs and settings, it is more likely for a research claim to be false than true.

---

[9] https://journals.plos.org/plosmedicine/article?id=10.1371/journal.pmed.0020124

Moreover, for many current scientific fields, claimed research findings may often be simply accurate measures of the prevailing bias. In this essay, I discuss the implications of these problems for the conduct and interpretation of research.

Breaking that down a bit, most studies were too small or too easily fudged (usually accidentally) to yield reliable results. Since this report many journals have taken steps to minimize the problem, such as requiring scientists to declare ahead of time what the experiment is about, and to share their data. But aside from inadvertent bias and small study size, something good and expected is happening to make most single studies "wrong".

You don't put a lot of research dollars into a study until you have a pretty good idea that it's worth doing. Think of that as building a railroad. You want a good idea of what's happening beyond that next range of hills before you start laying track. So you send out smaller teams to explore the landscape. Many are going to come back and report that it's no good building in that direction, while a few might come back with a good route.

Small studies are how you explore at the frontier of science. With less at risk you can give something a try and get a sense if there's something there or not. After enough encouraging preliminary studies you might call for a higher-powered, more rigorous (and expensive) experiment.

Nobody complains if the explorers come back and say "don't build down this valley" because they've saved you from an expensive mistake. And the small, single studies that serve as explorers are, by their nature, more likely to find those impassible valleys.

Here's another way to appreciate science being self-correcting: Airplanes spend most of their time off course. The last time you were on an airliner, most of the time it wasn't where it was supposed to be, or even pointing in exactly the right direction. And, yet, you got to your destination just fine. Why? Because navigating an airplane is also a self-correcting process. The navigation equipment and the pilots know which way to turn because something has told them to make a correction. These days, of course, airliners spend all of their time *really close* to the right course, and are pointed *almost* exactly the right direction. The corrections are so small that you never notice them, but if you had a way of precisely following the plane's track through the sky you'd see every little wobble. Computers have made the wobbles smaller, but they're still there.

OK, so what has this to do with your food? Plenty. There is no end of unscrupulous marketers willing to frighten or impress you with the "latest science" in order to sell you something you don't need, or which could actually hurt you. When radioactivity was first identified, and was the "latest science", there were people literally selling radium to eat and drink. Since there are small, single studies coming up with all kinds of results, these scammers can latch onto one they like, wrap their marketing in some sciency-sounding verbiage and sell you some snake oil.

Even when that doesn't happen, there's the problem of bad science reporting in the media. Most news outlets don't even have science reporters anymore, and even those that do often make mistakes. They like sensational stories. That's another term for click bait.

If you chase after "the latest study" while making dietary decisions you're likely basing your choice on an incorrect study, one that doesn't have the power or design to make any useful predictions let alone lifestyle advice. Stick with the consensus.

Now, I love following science news and hope you do, too. It's fine to read about the latest work because what scientists do is exciting and interesting. But don't mistake exploration at the frontiers of science for a solid consensus.

And then there's the whole mouse problem.

Of Mice and Men

For reasons ethical, economic, and more, doing experiments on people is difficult and expensive. You can't just starve half of your study group to see what happens. So tests on people are done rather late in the research process. A very common stand-in is the lab rat, or the lab mouse. They breed quickly, work cheaply, and can be extremely helpful in those early, exploratory kinds of experiments. A lot of work is done on mice.

That's why you see a lot of news stories breathlessly touting some kind of miraculous medical breakthrough — in mice. Again, this is usually fascinating stuff, but the last few decades have made something very clear: Mice are not people.

Who knew, right?

Extrapolating results from mice to humans is nearly impossible. The only way to make the connection is to cautiously move from those to other experiments and eventually to human trials. This takes years — even decades — to do. Today's actual, valid, lifesaving medical breakthrough might have been a mouse trial twenty years ago. So when you see a story about studies on mice, go ahead and cheer on the scientists, but do not make any changes to your diet or lifestyle based on it.

Keep in mind that nutritional science is extremely complicated. Nutrition studies tend to be observational and longitudinal. That means slow, expensive, and messy. It's really best to wait for a consensus to emerge.

And the consensus is what I've worked very hard to base this book on.

If Your Diet Has a Name It's Probably Bogus

Food fads are also driven mostly by fear, and specifically fear of modernity. I already mentioned the MSG scare and the gluten-free fad. Note that avoiding gluten is not a mere fad for people with Celiac Disease. They never say things like, "I just feel better when I skip the bagel." Even a little gluten can cause them serious, uncomfortable distress. As for those who claim that there's such a thing as NCGS, or Non Celiac Gluten Sensitivity, the science is not settled on that yet. The most recent information of which I am aware is that it's looking like it's not a thing, rather a misinterpretation of something else such as FODMAPS sensitivity.[10] But until we have a solid scientific consensus the best we can say is that Celiac is likely the only reason anybody needs to avoid gluten. For most of the world it's a healthy protein that gives baked goods structure. You could argue that civilization was built on gluten. There's nothing inherently wrong with it. Products are not better, healthier, or more "natural" just for being gluten-free.

---

[10]https://www.sciencemag.org/news/2018/05/what-s-really-behind-gluten-sensitivity

When you list food fads that nakedly appeal to a fear of modernity and a longing for bygone days when things were more "natural" it's hard to beat the Paleo Diet. This food fad posits a number of absurd things. Let's look at them one at a time.

We evolved to eat the diet of our Paleolithic ancestors. Do tell. Exactly which diet would that be? By the Paleolithic era there were humans all over the globe, eating all kinds of different diets. In fact, we only have a dim idea of what any of those Paleolithic diets actually consisted of. And what makes the Paleolithic special anyway? Did evolution stop there for some reason? Don't think so.

Paleolithic food was healthier. Healthier how? We already know that it's impossible to call one food healthier than another, but some diets can have better or worse outcomes than others. It's not clear exactly what paleo faddists think happened to food since then, but apparently getting more modern is somehow a bad thing.

Paleolithic people led healthier lives. Pull the other one. One reason ancient peoples had to start popping out babies as teenagers is that few children survived to adulthood and those who did rarely survived to be grandparents. Out in nature pretty much everything is trying to kill you. Nature is pretty good at this, having had eons of practice. It's really only in the last very few centuries — a blink in evolutionary time — that humans have turned the tables on nature in any significant way.

It's incandescently obvious that the Paleo Diet is just an Appeal to Antiquity.[11] That's far from the only problem with it. Even if we did manage to learn what foods a particular tribe of Paleolithic ancestors ate, we wouldn't be able to follow in their gustatory footsteps *because the ingredients don't exist anymore.* If a paleo proponent tells you that a hot dog is paleo, ask them how far back they think hot dog technology goes. (Sausages go back to perhaps the 13th century, and hot dogs as we know them are barely more than a century old.)[12] The very first domestication of cattle even remotely resembling beef happened about 10,000 years ago. Oops, that's just at or after the end of the Paleolithic.

---

[11] http://www.logicalfallacies.info/relevance/appeals/appeal-to-tradition/
[12] https://en.wikipedia.org/wiki/Hot_dog#History

This is the kind of absurdity you reach when you don't take evolution into account. We have evolved since then, *and so has our food.* Once agriculture got traction, we started accelerating the evolution of everything we eat. Today we can do the same thing but quicker, better, and safer using precision genetic engineering tools. But we have always changed our food. Nothing much that our stone age progenitors munched on is even available for us. Nary a single item that a Paleo enthusiast insists is actually Paleo even existed during the Paleolithic era. The rules are so arbitrary that I like to say you can easily eat Paleo if you just imagine a cave man gnawing on whatever you're about to eat. Presto! It's Paleo! Paleo pancakes, anyone?

There's another red flag associated with the Paleo diet, one that extends to every other fad diet you can name.

It has a name.

Why should that be a problem? Because, often, people name things when they invent them. So just about every diet with a name was invented by someone. Why should *that* be a problem? In nearly all cases, this invention happened with inadequate if not zero science. It was just someone's idea. Everybody knows how to eat, so everybody thinks they're an expert on food.

We need to take a side trip into the land of *It Worked For Me.* Those four words have misled more people than possibly any other simple statement in human history. It's how we fool ourselves, and it's exactly why science had to be invented. Personal experience is a very powerful teacher. Too powerful, it turns out. When our favorite team wins on a day when we wore their jersey it primes us to think that the jersey was responsible. Then we wear the shirt again on game days and a very interesting thing happens: We remember the wins, and not the losses. In other words, we remember the days when our team won while we were wearing the colors, and forget the days that they lost. Similarly, we remember the days they lost when we neglected our team-boosting attire and forget the days when they lost even though we wore our "lucky jersey". The name for this phenomenon is Confirmation Bias.[13]

This is exactly how the MSG scare happened. That one article primed people to think that "MSG sensitivity" was a thing. Any time they felt a

---

[13] https://en.wikipedia.org/wiki/Confirmation_bias

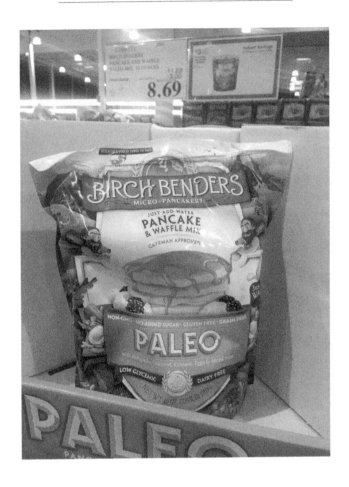

little odd after some Chinese food then, by golly, it had to be the MSG that did it. If they ate something later with tomato and Parmesan cheese (both of which naturally contain MSG) they didn't notice that they felt fine. This is also how all *So-Called Alternative Medicine*, or SCAM, works. All of it.

You know what? The more I learn about confirmation bias the more I see it everywhere.

Everybody has confirmation bias. No exceptions. It's just how we're built. So if we want to learn how the world actually works, what can we do? We can use a systematic method for observing nature, and apply consistent logic to evaluate the results. That means taking careful observations which become real data, then trying to prove ourselves wrong. If we fail to prove an idea wrong then we get other people to try to prove it wrong. Any idea that survives that can provisionally be considered to be correct.

There's a name for this method: *science*. That's all science is. Dr. Steven Novella, a neurologist and noted skeptic, put it well:

> "What do you think science is? There is nothing magical about science. It is simply a systematic way for carefully and thoroughly observing nature and using consistent logic to evaluate results. So which part of that exactly do you disagree with? Do you disagree with being thorough? Using careful observation? Being systematic? Or using consistent logic?"

So "It worked for me" is simply an expression of our confirmation bias. We can't know what effect a food or ingredient has on us by just trying some and seeing what happens. Of course, if we happen to be allergic that can be a different story. Even then it usually takes careful tests to find out exactly what, if anything, we're allergic or intolerant to. It's so easy to incorrectly believe that you have a food allergy that a survey found nearly 40% of Americans believe they have one, when the reality is closer to 10%.[14] So three out of four people who think they have a food allergy don't have one at all.

Another natural part of human nature is to think that if something works for us that it will work for everybody. So everyone who has lost weight or improved their health thinks that what they did is the right thing for everybody else. Instantly they're an expert! And some people come at the problem as orthorexics who just invent rules about the right way to eat. Often as not these people have something to sell, and they set themselves up as health gurus.

---

[14] https://jamanetwork.com/journals/jamanetworkopen/fullarticle/2720064

Never trust a health guru.

Anne Hathaway, the glamorous and talented movie star, appeared in 2019 on the *Ellen* show to promote her latest film, *Serenity.* She told a story about how she and her family happened upon a "hippy enclave" where she learned a fascinating health secret. She had Ellen, and every member of the studio audience, check under their seats for the clementine that had been placed there. Everyone was asked to peel it and place the whole fruit in their mouth while Anne explained the wonders of "citrus healing", a method for incorporating citrus into your meditation. She called it "clementime".

And then she told everybody the truth: She had made the whole thing up. "The takeaway of this is: Do not put something in your mouth just because a celebrity tells you to. You are free to throw your clementine at me now."

I love Anne Hathaway for many reasons, but mostly for doing this.

You don't need a guru, and nobody who understands how nutrition actually works would set themselves up as one, nor try to sell anything as The Right Diet. There is no one "right" diet. Remember that we are omnivores, evolved to thrive on a variety of diets. We can happily eat our way around the planet, and we have.

I do not want to be your diet guru. You will note that I eschew hard and fast rules. I've already admitted that I could be wrong about something. If and when the scientific consensus changes, go with that. If your medical doctor tells you that you need to change your diet, change it. Never change the way you eat just because some "guru", even a famous or glamorous one, said so. Because when they say, "It worked for me" your response should always be, "That's nice. How do you know?"

As a simple heuristic, if you treat every diet that has a name as being bogus you will be right far more often than you are wrong. Don't get hung up looking for an "ideal" diet. It doesn't exist.

Now that we know where food fads come from we should just be able to ignore them. But a few are currently so prevalent that they're worth enumerating. I already mentioned how, for non-Celiacs, "Gluten Free" is pretty much a fad. We also covered the poster child for fear of modernity, Paleo. Let's take a gander at a few other current fads.

Keto (or Ketogenic)

This is a very deep rabbit hole, enough for a series of blog posts by Anthony Warner, the Angry Chef. If you're curious about details I encourage you to read them. A short one is here,[15] and a longer series is here.[16] The tl;dr is that ketosis is a state the body can get into when there's insufficient glucose. Remember that your body prefers to run on glucose. Running out of it is a bad thing, as anybody who has observed a type 1 diabetic in hypoglycemia can attest. The Angry Chef sums it up well:

> The body only has very limited stores of glucose, so during starvation, when a lack of nutrition might easily cause our blood sugar to drop, it sometimes uses a clever fall back mechanism to prevent blood glucose falling too low. It can flip a metabolic switch and enter a state of ketosis, delivering ketone bodies derived from fat into the bloodstream, and allowing the brain, muscles and other organs to use them as an alternative fuel. This switch decreases the amount of glucose our body uses, meaning that an optimum blood level can be maintained for longer, very useful in staving off coma and death if we have to go without food.

So why would people deliberately want to trigger a starvation response? Longing for that magic bullet, and a misunderstanding of the science. There are claims that keto can help with a lot of things, but there are only small, preliminary studies to back that up.[17] No consensus yet.

It turns out that a ketogenic diet used to be prescribed for treating epileptic children. This is pretty much no longer the case but, apparently to some people, if it's good for epileptic children then it must be good for everybody. Remember that thing about broken legs and crutches? Even if it turns out that ketosis can help with, say, diabetes, that doesn't mean that it's good for non-diabetics.

There's no scientific reason to induce ketosis no matter what kind of testimonials you see on the web, and there are plenty of reasons not

---

[15] https://www.bodyforwife.com/keto-is-the-dumbfuck-diet-cult-du-jour-but-that-wont-last/

[16] https://angry-chef.com/blog/the-natural-alternative-part-1

[17] https://skeptoid.com/episodes/4664

to try. Also note that most ketogenic diets lack variety because they concentrate on just fats and proteins. There are potential side effects, some of which could be serious. The worst thing would be to delay or avoid actual medical treatment by using the Keto diet instead.

If your doctor has you on a ketogenic diet for a medically valid reason, stick with it. Otherwise, it's probably best to treat it as a fad and give it a pass.

Mediterranean Diet

Arguably the least bogus of the named fads, it shares one problem with the Paleo diet: There isn't a single Mediterranean diet. That name really traces back to a specific diet that was tested in a weight loss program, but now refers, rather vaguely, to the way people eat in several different cultures around the Mediterranean. You will find claims that it is the "world's healthiest diet". Yet we now know that there is no one "healthiest diet". Many diets that could be called Mediterranean are, however, perfectly healthy ones. They feature legumes, fresh produce, and the like. You could even describe them as, oh, I don't know, a variety of foods, mostly plants, with plenty of veggies and fruits, not too much or too little.

Alkaline Diet

Some claim that certain foods or kinds of water can "correct" the alkalinity of your body. This is, to be blunt, dangerous flapdoodle. Your body tightly regulates the pH (acidity/alkalinity) of your blood. If something you ate actually did change your body's alkalinity you'd end up in one of two places: an ambulance or a hearse.

Fruitarianism

A common human failing is thinking that "if a little is good, more is better". Fruitarians take the fact that fruit is healthy and extrapolate it to *only* fruit is healthy. Obviously that would narrow your diet quite a bit, and if you ate only fruit you'd be missing out on many vital nutrients.

Never go with a diet that has extreme ideas about eating *only* this or *never* eating that.

Blood Type Diet

This one is just nuts. The claim is that your blood type determines what your ideal diet should be. There isn't an iota of science to back up this claim, of course. It's just an assertion made by people who think they've found The Secret. What is true is that there is a tiny amount of pre-liminary science (namely one encouraging study) indicating that maybe, someday, we'll be able to get personalized diet recommendations based on a series of lab tests. The odds that blood type will be part of those tests are vanishingly small.

I could go on and on. Fortunately Wikipedia has already gone on and on for me. You can look up a list of fad diets[18] there and rest assured that they're all likely bogus to one degree or another.

Let's Go to the Store

Enough about how *not* to eat. We've left behind the fear, the gurus, and the fads. We know that a healthy diet is a variety of foods, mostly plants, with plenty of vegetables and fruits, not too much or too little.

Now we stand in the grocery store amid bewildering plenty and decide what's for dinner.

Let's start in the produce section, shall we? In many American super-markets this is a sadly vestigial section that isn't nearly as big as it should be. But it's there that we'll find what should, on average, make up a major portion of our diet: fruits and vegetables. You knew before you bought this book that you should be eating fruits and veggies, right? There are many reasons for this, including vitamins and fiber, but let's just go with our guiding principal of variety.

Take a look around. Each bin has a different species of food in it. There are root vegetables, leafy greens, tubers, and all manner of fruits and veggies. Take in the view with all its pretty colors and varied textures.

---

[18]https://en.wikipedia.org/wiki/Fad_diet#List_of_fad_diets

Then let's make a little detour to the snack aisle. Look at all the brightly colored boxes and bags. Check the ingredients.

Here's the main thing you need to know about ingredient lists: They're listed by order of weight. The first ingredient on the list is the main one, and at the end of the list are typically things that come in vanishingly small quantities, such as coloring or preservatives. Remember how *-ose* chemicals are all sugars? You'll sometimes see multiple sugars listed separately in hopes that you won't recognize them. That's OK, because sugars get totaled in the Nutrition Facts part of the label. (That's the American system. Most countries have something similar enough.)

Back to the stuff in the snack aisle. That's mostly wheat, corn, or potatoes as the main ingredients. You'll probably see fats high on the list as well.

There's nothing at all wrong with wheat, corn, and potatoes. And any of those efficiently-marketed and precision-engineered foods can, of course, be part of your healthy diet. Just not a major part. You get no variety points for having three different kinds of crackers and five flavors of potato chips. Turn around again and head back to that produce section.

That's more like it, isn't it? Oh, look: There is even corn (on the cob) and potatoes. Wander over and check out the potatoes for a minute. Hey, there are multiple species of *potato* here! Potatoes are awesome. Russets for baking, Yukon Golds for mashing or hashing, even little red ones for roasting. Sidle on over to the leafy greens. How many species of lettuce do you see? Even in a relatively sad grocery store there are usually several. Check out the tomatoes. Again, probably several kinds. Squash? Heavens! So many squashes. Mushrooms? Why, there must be at least—

Wait a minute. Are mushrooms vegetables? No. Actually they're closer to being animals than plants. (You should find a book about fungi. They're amazing.) But, culinarily, go ahead and treat them like vegetables. You can rack up lots of variety points with different mushroom species. If you're just learning to cook, mushrooms are like having a superpower. Know why? They're made of chitin (say KITE-in), the same protein that crabs use to make their shells. What that means is that *you can't overcook mushrooms*. How cool is that? Strap on that apron, maybe put a little oil in a heavy pan, toss in sliced mushrooms, crank the soundtrack to *Ratatouille*, and go to town. You can't mess them up unless the heat is so high that they burn. They just get more and more concentrated, ready to bring some umami goodness to whatever you're making. And you can eat most of them raw, if you'd rather.

More on cooking later. Let's continue our tour. Check out the carrots, sweet, orange, and sexy. You can peel, slice or shred them to enjoy raw, you can steam them, you can cook them, roast them, even grill them. You can even buy so-called baby carrots in a bag if you're feeling lazy. But they aren't really babies. They're just whittled down from longer, skinnier carrots. There's crunchy celery. Ooh — over there are broccoli and Brussels sprouts. (Oh, yeah. If you think you don't like them, you just haven't had them done right. We'll fix that in the *Joy of Food* chapter.) Those bright bell peppers are aching to add tantalizing color to a salad.

Know what? Make it a point the next time you go to the store to explore the entire produce department. Look at every single thing there. Take a moment to be glad you aren't one of your Paleolithic ancestors, scrounging for food while avoiding predators. Your biggest worry right now is getting your shopping cart past that guy who is blocking aisle 5, bewildered by all the olive oil choices.

Here's a fun game: I'm fortunate to live close to one of the best grocery stores in the country. The produce section is as big as many entire grocery stores. There are vegetables there that are complete mysteries to me. So my game is to pick a vegetable I've never heard of, buy it, and learn how to prepare it. It's easy to find recipes on line, and don't forget to ask the grocer who stocks the place for tips. They typically know their stuff.

There's more to the store, of course. There are lentils, beans, nuts, seeds. There are chickpeas, the lentil that can't decide if it's a pea, a bean (garbanzo), or a gram. Many kinds of olives, if you're lucky. Breads, cereals, meats, fish. You can, of course, find dairy products such as milk, cheese, and butter. All groovy, as long as you aren't lactose intolerant, but note that dairy products all add up to only one measly species variety point. Moo.

Let's swing by the frozen section. I want to show you something. See those frozen peas? They're actually better than the "fresh" ones you might have seen (but probably didn't) over in the produce aisle. Why? Science! The technology of flash freezing allows them to be harvested and frozen incredibly quickly. Many foods, including peas and corn, begin to lose their sweetness and texture within minutes of being harvested. In this case, "frozen at the peak of freshness" is more than mere marketing lingo.

As long as we're here, there are plenty of frozen fruits and veggies to choose from. Highly convenient, to boot. Oh, and if you've been particularly good then your store has frozen *wild* blueberries. They're a very different animal than the plump, blue, domesticated ones. Try them in baking. Oh, yum.

Further down the aisle is the ice cream. Really yummy, but only two variety points (dairy and sugar) to speak of. Maybe save that for special occasions. Or, when you have a hankering for ice cream, maybe go to an ice cream specialty store to make an occasion of it. And look, there's the frozen pizza.

Don't giggle. Take a look at the Nutrition Facts on a few. You may be surprised. There are some small, thin-crust ones that are 2 "servings" of only 350 calories each. Yeah, so you could chow down on the whole pizza and have a very reasonably-sized meal of 700 calories. Every now and then. Remember, there aren't many variety points to be had with a typical pizza. It's mostly wheat and dairy fat.

As you wander the store just remember that ingredients are listed in order of their weight in each food product. Things are mostly made of the two or three items at the top of the list, and have teensy amounts of the things at the end of the list. So pay the most attention to the first ingredients when deciding how much variety you're getting and how much of this food should be part of your healthy diet. If you wander back to that snack aisle and peep the labels on a few more things you'll see exactly what I mean. Feel free to snort derisively if an ingredient featured on the front of the box is way down the list. But don't let that stop you from enjoying whatever it is — if you like it and don't overdo it.

Oh, there's the drink aisle. That's a lot of sugar and water. I don't know about you, but I'd rather get my ration of sugar from better stuff than that. Sure, you can treat yourself now and then to a sugary drink, but don't drink it or buy it by the liter. And if you really have to have some, see if there's a sugar-free version.

So go ahead and load up the cart with lovely food to take home. Note how anything labeled "organic" is likely more expensive. You can skip that stuff entirely, knowing that you're not only saving money but helping the environment. That's a lot better than shopping out of fear, isn't it?

Later in the book we'll talk about preparing all of this lovely food. For now I just want you to see your local grocery store with freshly educated, fear-free eyes.

Chapter 5

How to Lose Weight Safely

Who should lose weight?

Before digging into the topic of weight loss we have to answer a basic, vital question: Who should lose weight? Maybe you should, and maybe you shouldn't. There is no one ideal weight for anybody. We all have a range of healthy weights, and as close to ideal as you can get is to be somewhere near the lean end of that range. While obesity increases the risks of many negative health outcomes, just being overweight isn't nearly as bad for you as the scolds would have you believe.

If you are considering making a big change in your weight, start by talking to your medical doctor. Find out how far out of your healthy range you actually are, if at all. Don't use unrealistic metrics or expectations. And by unrealistic I mostly mean models, actors, and celebrities. Pictures in magazines are perhaps the worst guide. In many cases the bodies you see there aren't even human — they've been sculpted using Photoshop. Let health, not vanity, be your guide.

Speaking of expectations…

Unless you are their doctor, what another person weighs or how they eat is none of your business. Keep your opinions to yourself.

A theme of this book is that personal tastes, and matters of health, should never be treated as issues of right and wrong, good and evil. It's simply not a moral question, and a huge cause of unhealthy relationships with food is forgetting this and heaping righteous scorn on people who we think are dong it wrong. (The target of this ire is sometimes ourselves, about which more later.)

But it's not our affair. We need to stay out of it. Don't comment on another person's weight. Don't comment on how they eat, how much they eat, or what they eat. Not directly, not passive-aggressively, not even dropping hints or rolling eyes. You have enough to do just taking care of yourself.

Parents: Never, *ever* comment on your child's weight. Don't tell them they're skinny. In the name of all that is holy *never* tell them they're fat. Really. Just don't do it. It could kill them. Think I'm exaggerating? Talk to people who have survived and recovered from an eating disorder. A nickel says you'll hear stories of a mom or a dad, perhaps even well-meaning, telling them they're fat. Or that they should drop a few pounds. If you have any concern about your child's weight, either too heavy or too light, *discuss it with their doctor* and let the doctor decide what, if anything, to tell them. Eating disorders are the deadliest mental illness there is. Don't mess with them.

Similarly, don't comment on how much your child eats. Don't criticize them for what they eat. Do provide a healthy diet in the home. Do avoid stocking the house with snacks that should really be rare treats. But chill. Perhaps you've forgotten what it was like to eat as a teenager. Boys, in particular, can put away astonishing amounts of food. So can girls sometimes. That's fine. They're growing, they're active, and their metabolisms are at a lifetime high. Smile, take a deep breath, and make a few extra pancakes.

Teens (and younger children) should not lose weight except under direct medical supervision.

This is really important. *A healthy child is constantly gaining weight.* That's called growing. It's quite common for some kids to go through a pudgy phase and then grow into their weight. Anybody's weight will fluctuate, and kids can be all over the map. As I said above, you do *not* want to even slightly increase the risk of an eating disorder.

Something almost all eating disorders have in common is being an unhealthy coping mechanism for stress. By stress I mean feelings of helplessness and being out of control. These feelings can be greatly amplified in people under 25 years of age, in part because the judgement center in their prefrontal cortex has not yet fully developed. Food restrictions can appear to them to be "something I can control". That's a very dangerous road. I'll talk more about eating disorders and how to deal with them in a later chapter. For now I just want to raise the red flag that weight loss at a young age is fraught with risk.

Nobody under 20 years of age should ever attempt to lose weight except under the direct supervision of a medical doctor. And most people over that age should check with their doctor first anyway.

So say you and your doctor have agreed that you need to shed a kilo or two. Let's look at some considerations when choosing a goal weight, and then at weight loss itself.

How Much Should You Weigh?

This is not a weight loss book. It certainly isn't a diet book, where diet is used as a verb. But that won't stop us from covering pretty much everything you need to know about it, all in a single chapter. It's hard to picture a field more packed with misinformation, ripoffs, and fear than weight loss. Women, in particular, are targeted by the so-called "wellness" and weight loss industries. It is, as the expression goes, a target rich environment. Let's start by laying out out a few basic precepts.

There are exactly two ways to lose weight:

1. Surgery
2. A sustained calorie deficit

That's it. If you want to lose weight you either pay someone, hopefully a doctor, to remove some part of your body, or you maintain a calorie deficit. There are no other choices. Many weight loss surgeries, such as gastric banding, are just ways of getting someone to that calorie deficit. Liposuction is an example of a surgery that simply removes the fat from the body. Surgery for weight loss is typically a last-ditch effort that a doctor will only recommend to people who are severely overweight and in significant danger. If you are in that condition you need to put down this book and call the doctor anyway.

Your body can store food energy for later use. That's what it does most of the time when it converts food energy into fat. This is how we survived as a species through famines and winters. Fat is also an insulator that helps keep you warm, and serves other functions in the body. You need some fat on you. For almost all of human history there has barely or rarely been enough food. That's why we evolved this storage mechanism. In much of the developed world we now enjoy such an amazing abundance that it's all too easy to maintain a year-round, sustained calorie *surplus*. That, of course, is how weight gain happens. The only other way a mature adult can gain weight is by adding muscle mass. This is generally considered a good kind of weight gain. It means you're getting plenty of exercise. Muscle protects you from injury and, as a bonus, it raises your metabolism a little bit.

A calorie is a calorie.

At least when you're actually talking about calories. A calorie is a unit of heat energy. It's the amount of heat required to raise the temperature of 1 gram of water by 1 degree Celsius at 1 atmosphere of pressure. Oh, wait. That's the *small calorie*. When we see Calories listed on foods in America we're really looking at kilocalories, or *kcal*. Some labels, especially in Europe, actually say kcal. That's so that we don't have to juggle big numbers, like an apple having 90,000 calories. Much nicer to say 90 kcal and, in America, we just say 90 Calories. Except for this paragraph or where noted otherwise, all references to calories in this book are the convenient "big" calories, or *kcal*.

It may seem odd to measure the energy in food with heat, but think about it a minute. Ever heard of someone assuming room temperature? Yes, we are exothermic machines. Everything we do generates heat. And that energy has to come from somewhere.

The most common way to measure the caloric content of a food ingredient is to set it on fire and examine the heat you get out. That's just a faster version of what your body is doing, namely combining chemicals with oxygen to release energy. That's why the metaphor of "burning" calories is apt. We even get the same chemical outputs as combustion: water and carbon dioxide. In case you ever wondered where fat goes when you lose weight, it exits mostly via exhaling CO_2 and urinating water.

Clever you! I know what you're thinking! If it takes calories to warm water up, I could lose weight by drinking cold water! In fact, you'll probably hear that idea out there on the internet. It's absolutely true that it takes calories to warm up water.

You know there's a "but" coming. Here it is. Warming an ice-cold glass of water up to body temperature uses a little under (drum roll, please) 4 calories. Oh, well. It was a spiffy idea, and it means you understand what calories actually are. Next time you have ice cream you can smile like a sage knowing that your body will melt that sweet treat in your stomach using the energy in a tiny fraction of your first spoonful. Pretty marvelous, when you think about it.

Some readers have made it this far and are still fuming at "a calorie is a calorie". Thanks for sticking with me. A calorie wouldn't be a useful scientific measurement if it magically changed now and then. *The ways we get calories from different foods, though, are very different.* There's a lot of complicated chemistry at work, and the body handles different kinds of foods differently. This still doesn't make any food fattening, but it's worth understanding that different foods have different short and long term effects, including in how your body reaps and squirrels away calories from them. What matters for weight loss is your long term calorie balance, not where the calories come from. This is a game of diets, not foods, and of weeks and months, not hours and days.

For our purposes in this chapter, just lose the idea that there are "good calories" and "bad calories". In the long run, for our purposes here, there are only calories. We'll talk about the differences between foods in detail elsewhere, as it really doesn't make much difference in the context of weight loss.

So how much should you weigh?

There is no one ideal weight for anybody. We all have a range of healthy weights, and most doctors and nutrition scientists want to see you aim for somewhere on the lean end of that range. But weight alone is not a good predictor of health outcomes. In fact, you should always be suspicious when someone tries to boil something as complicated as health down to a single number.

Speaking of deceptive single numbers, just ignore your BMI. The Body Mass Index[1] was developed to help simply describe populations of people. It's a single number derived from the mass, or weight, and height of an individual, specifically the body mass divided by the square of the body height. The important thing to note is that it only takes two numbers as its input: your height and your weight. It does not account for your muscle mass versus your fat. This means that fit, muscular people can have a high BMI while clearly not being overweight. Let's use the example of someone that just about everybody has seen many times, president George W. Bush. Whatever else you think of him, you'd never call him fat. But his BMI put him in the "overweight" category.

Your doctor may find your BMI to be a useful part of a diagnosis, typically on the lower end when evaluating you for an eating disorder. Aside from that, while it may say things about populations that are useful to epidemiologists, *BMI says almost nothing useful about an individual.*[2]

Waist circumference is actually closer to being a useful single number than just about anything else. Very roughly speaking, if your waist isn't noticeably bigger than your hips then you're probably OK. As always, if you have reason to be concerned about your weight you should consult your doctor, who can help determine what a healthy weight for you would be and how far you are from it, if at all.

If you and your doctor have determined that you should lose weight, read on. And please promise me that if your doctor suggests something different than what I do that you'll listen to the doctor. At least assuming your doctor isn't one of those who has gone off the rails on diet. More about those doctors later in the book.

First let's look at safe ways to lose weight, or in other words maintain that moderate calorie deficit, and at how to spot scams and dangerous weight loss advice.

---

[1] https://en.wikipedia.org/wiki/Body_mass_index
[2] https://www.popsci.com/better-than-BMI

Don't Diet

Never go on a diet. Diets don't work.

That sounds like quite a claim. For an in depth look at why it's true, read the excellent book *Secrets From the Eating Lab: The Science of Weight Loss, the Myth of Willpower, and Why You Should Never Diet Again*[3] by Traci Mann. The basic ideas are simple.

I have to pause here to point out that the word *diet* is rather overloaded. Your diet, the noun, which describes the totality of what and how you eat, is not what we're discussing in this chapter. I mean diet, the verb, meaning some change you make to the way you eat in order to lose weight.

Dieting, or temporarily restricting/changing your diet is, rather obviously, *temporary*. It makes no sense at all to expect long term results from a temporary effort. Any diet that results in a calorie deficit will make you lose weight. And then if you go back to eating the way you used to, guess what. You'll go right back to your old weight, if not higher. You have to permanently change the way you eat and live your life if you want to stay at your goal weight. But it's best to make the change as the way to get *to* that goal weight.

There are no silver bullets. There are no hacks. There are no cheats, pills, potions, elixirs, supplements, exercises, or diets that will change any of that. It's very simple: Eat a diet that's in calorie balance, or your weight will change.

Note that simple does not mean easy. For some people nature and circumstances conspire to make losing weight and keeping it off very difficult. But it is *possible* for everybody, because there are no loopholes in the laws of thermodynamics. There's no reason to make it more difficult by chasing ideas that don't work or, worse, make you heavier or sicker.

Don't rely on willpower.

That's a recipe for failure. It's covered in detail in Traci Mann's book, mentioned above, but the idea is pretty simple: Willpower isn't really a

---

[3] *Secrets From the Eating Lab: The Science of Weight Loss, the Myth of Willpower, and Why You Should Never Diet Again*

thing. The cognitive load of keeping yourself in a constant state of denial or sacrifice is fatiguing. You will give up, you will go back to living the way you used to, and the weight will come back.

Have a treat day, not a cheat day.

Take a moment to consider a fad diet that uses vocabulary like "cheat day". See how there's an implication that you're doing something *wrong*, and maybe getting away with it? That's an orthorexic attitude right there, isn't it? But when you're eating a healthy diet you're certainly allowed an occasional *treat day* because, as we've seen, what you eat today doesn't matter, while what you eat this month (ie: longer term) does. And *treat* is a much healthier idea than cheat!

Take your time.

It's extremely rare for rapid weight loss to not go wrong. It increases your risk of developing an eating disorder, which can literally be deadly. More typically you will rebound, ending up weighing more than you did when you started. It's worse to have your weight dramatically yo-yo than to just be overweight and stable.

It's time to meet your BMR, or Basal Metabolic Rate. This is essentially the number of calories per day that you need just to stay alive. Imagine that you were bedridden 24/7 with no chance for exercise. Getting your BMR worth of calories would just keep you alive and at your current weight. This isn't a number that you need to know with any great precision, and the estimates you get from on line calculators such as the one at bmi-calculator.net[4] are quite adequate. The main thing to remember is never to eat less than your BMR for more than a day or two. In other words, if your weight loss plan has a daily calorie budget less than your BMR, it's too aggressive. You are, at that point, essentially starving yourself for no good reason.

Many people understandably confuse BMR with TDEE, or Total Daily Energy Expenditure. That's the total number of calories you burn

---

[4]http://www.bmi-calculator.net/bmr-calculator/

in a day of typical activity. You can get a very rough, close-enough-for-rock-and-roll estimate using a TDEE calculator[5] or any one of a number of diet-oriented apps. Again, forget precision. This is horse shoes and hand grenades, not archery. When calculating a calorie deficit, should you choose to count calories, you start with the TDEE and subtract the goal deficit. Never start by subtracting from your BMR because that won't get you enough food.

You can safely lose up to approximately 2 pounds, or 1 kilo, per week. That's the fastest you should plan on. I don't care if you have a wedding or a big date coming up in two weeks, don't try to go faster than this. If you're smart (and you are, because you're reading this book) you'll aim for something more like half that, or 1 pound (half kilo) per week.

There are multiple reasons why that's a winning strategy. First, it's just easier and more comfortable. Who doesn't like easy and comfortable? Second, it's healthier and safer. Last, but not least, it increases your odds of being able to keep the weight off when you reach your goal. Consider dropping that rate to half a pound (quarter kilo) per week when you get within a few pounds of your goal. It makes the transition to a maintenance diet almost effortless.

And there is never, ever, a reason to hurry. If you're 50 pounds overweight, a year is a perfectly reasonable time to spend reaching your goal weight. Ignore promises of several pounds per week. Those tabloid diets usually reduce water weight more than fat anyway. And they are a bad idea because they're unhealthy, too fast, and well, because they're diets. Remember: *never* diet.

It takes about 3500 calories to build a pound of fat. Not a precise number, obviously, but close enough for our purposes. If you chose to count calories (more on that later, because maybe you shouldn't) you could use the rule of thumb that you aim for no more than a 500 calorie per day deficit. It should, I hope, be obvious that these approximations don't take into account your individual body composition, age, weight, activity, or hormonal levels. As I talk about elsewhere in the book, fine tuning is a loser's game. Close enough is good enough in this context.

---

[5] https://tdeecalculator.net/

Don't exercise to lose weight.

Calm down. I'm not telling you not to exercise. You should make regular exercise a part of your life. The benefits are amazingly wide-ranging and backed by more and more science every day. But if your goal is weight loss you should not start working out to lose weight. Why? Let's back up a bit. Remember our exhaustive list of things that cause weight loss? (I'll wait if you want to head back to the beginning of the chapter to check.) Notice what's not on that list? That's right, exercise.

Exercise does, of course, burn calories. And burning calories certainly *can* contribute to a sustained calorie deficit. There are some things about exercise that most people don't think about. One is that it burns a lot fewer calories than you probably think. There's a saying in the fitness world: You can't outrun your fork. Let's say you do high intensity calisthenics for about 30 minutes. That might burn on the order of roughly 250 calories. Nice workout! So you treat yourself to a Mango Pineapple Gatorade and a small granola bar. You know. For recovery. (More on that later, too.) That 8-ounce serving is 120 calories, and the bar is at least 100. See where this is going?

And you aren't likely to stop at that recovery snack. Exercise is also a very effective appetite enhancer, making you likely to eat more at your next meal than you would have. Psychologically you'll feel like you've "earned" a little extra, and those little extras add up quickly. People who jump into the gym and hit the weights hard on January 2nd often get discouraged when the pounds not only refuse to melt away (remember about not rushing it?) but may even keep piling on.

Psychologists talk about a phenomenon called moral licensing. This can apply to "slacktivism" where a sufficiently strongly worded Facebook post about your favorite issue gives you the same rewards as actually doing something about it, so you end up not actually doing something about it. A similar thing can happen with exercise, and even eating or drinking "diet" versions of food: It gives us license for a little extra treat.

You should exercise to be healthy, not to lose weight. While you are losing weight, don't add a lot of new exercise. This is another part of your strategy that you should consult the doctor about, partially to make sure your exercise regimen is safe. Do move around more. Take walks, get in the habit of using the stairs rather than the elevator when you can, but don't ramp up your workouts until you've reached or at least gotten close to your goal weight. At that point exercise really becomes your friend. People who keep the weight off long term tend to be those who exercise regularly. And do you know what their most common workout routine is? Walking.[6] But, as I mentioned before, the real key is a complete diet and lifestyle change. More on that soon.

This seems like a good time to point out that the body does not spot reduce. You'll see all sorts of fanciful claims about exercises to flatten your tummy, shrink your thighs, or even (I kid you not) target face fat.

Nope.

Your body is going to store fat where it wants to, and burn fat from where it wants to, and no exercise, cream, or magical food is going to change that. Exercise can target muscle groups for strength and mass, but not fat deposits.

There are no fattening foods.

You are not really what you eat. Eating fat doesn't make you fat, any more than gnawing on a carrot turns you into a root vegetable. Your body takes in nutrients, processes them into one of those seven things we talked about, throws away the stuff it doesn't want, uses what it can, and sometimes stores extra for a rainy day. It doesn't transform itself into what you ate.

Perhaps the most common way foods are demonized is by calling them fattening. There are no fattening foods. There are many fattening *diets*. In the context of weight, any diet with a sustained calorie surplus can cause fat gain, and usually does. On the other hand, you could lose weight eating any kind of food there is, as long as you maintain a sufficient calorie deficit. Yes, you could lose weight eating just doughnuts, pizza, or even plain butter. It wouldn't be a *healthy* diet, but it would be a *weight losing* diet.

Sometimes people call a food fattening when they really mean that it has a *high calorie density*. Animal fat is the densest, at around 9 calories

---

[6]https://www.self.com/story/i-lost-90-pounds-maintaining-that-weight-loss-was-harder

per gram. Straight sugar is a pretty calorie dense carbohydrate, clocking in at just under 3.9 calories per gram. A gram of celery, on the other hand, has such a low calorie density that a gram of it is legally 0 calories. You need to chew through an entire stalk of it to reach 6 calories. That doesn't make butter fattening, and it doesn't make celery a weight loss food. Different foods just have different calorie densities.

There are no foods, pills, supplements, or herbs that cause weight loss.

The market is awash in products claiming to "boost your metabolism", "melt away fat", or "promote weight loss"

Lies. All lies.

Did you see "eat special foods" on the exhaustive list of ways to lose weight? Neither did I, and I wrote it. Anybody selling you a "fat burner" is a scammer. It's a very human thing to look for a short cut, a secret trick, or a hack. There aren't any. Just as there are no fattening foods (just fattening diets) there are no slimming foods.

There are, of course, foods with a low calorie density. Those happen to mostly include the fruits and vegetables that you should be eating anyway.

There are, to be complete, prescription medications that a doctor might make part of a weight loss treatment. These don't work by "burning" fat or any such mumbo-jumbo. Their one goal is to make it easier to achieve that sustained calorie deficit. If your qualified medical doctor prescribes something, take it. But don't buy "diet pills" at retail.

Drink water for hydration, not weight loss.

Some people drink a lot of water before meal time as an appetite suppressant. Just having your stomach mechanically more full makes it harder for you to get more food in. This is actually a disordered behavior called *water loading*. It is not the sign of a healthy relationship with food, and it is not addressing the parts of your diet that matter. If you catch yourself doing this, skip ahead to the chapter *When Food Gets Scary*.

The nature of this book is that I have to spend a lot of time fighting common myths and misinformation, so you've noticed that it's heavy on the don'ts. Don't diet. Don't exercise to lose weight. When, oh when, I can hear you clamoring, do we get around to things we *should* do?

Now!

We have now established some ground rules:

- Weight loss requires a sustained calorie deficit.
- Keeping the weight off, and being healthy, requires a lifetime change in habits.
- A healthy diet consists of a variety of foods, mostly plants, including plenty of fruits and veggies.

So what we need to do next is change how we eat. It's mostly there in the third ground rule. There are as many ways to get a sustained calorie deficit as there are almonds on trees. There is no one best weight loss diet. If you're going to eat foods for the rest of your life, they should be foods you enjoy. There is no good reason to treat this as a punishment, and many good reasons not to. This is really an opportunity to look and feel better, live longer, and enjoy your life more.

Again, if you are making a significant change in your weight, start by consulting with your medical doctor. That's really important. Make sure you really do need to lose weight (you might be surprised) and, if so, how much. Make sure that nothing you do while losing weight jeopardizes another aspect of your health. So see the doctor, and then go slow.

You can, if you want, simply count calories. I do not recommend this for people who are easily obsessed or freaked out by numbers. There are apps which let you log all of your meals and calculate a calorie budget based on your weight goals. That's how I lost my last 40-ish pounds. Since I'm a geek, not triggered by numbers, and enjoy using apps, it worked fine for me. Beware, though: Many apps, including the one I used, Lose It![7], also promote some very sketchy ideas, such as DNA testing for weight loss (not a real thing, at least yet) or other such woo. If you use one, just use it to track calories and exercise. Ignore the sketchy stuff they're trying to sell you.

If, on the other hand, you never entertained yourself as a kid by counting the marbles in your bag or the ceiling tiles in your 4th Grade

---

[7] https://loseit.com/

classroom, you don't really need to do any counting at all. Because, even if you want to count calories, you still want to get the right variety of foods. So everybody can do this next part.

I said there are no hacks, but there are two simple tricks you can use to tune your diet toward a healthier one:

Eat your veggies first.

Repeated studies have shown that if you serve and eat your vegetable course first, you end up eating more vegetables. If you aren't in the habit of having vegetables first, when at home just serve that course first. As in don't bring anything else to the table until you finish the veggies. You don't have to make the servings any bigger, just have them first. More veggies in your diet not only makes the diet healthier (more varied) but lowers the calorie density of your diet.

Use simple barriers.

Building new habits is really a psychological problem. It turns out that it's not that hard to manipulate ourselves. For example, if you move a bowl of candy across the table to just out of reach, you'll eat less candy than if you leave it close to you. Having it far enough away that you have to get up and walk to it will cut consumption even further. So if there's a special treat food that's particularly attractive to you, just don't keep it in the house. Save it for special occasions. Like you have to leave the house to have any.

It's really about that simple. Put a little friction between you and the foods you want to cut back on. If you're a snacker, keep things like fruits close to hand. It can genuinely make a big difference.

For many people, simply cutting back on sweet snacks, avoiding sugary drinks, and dialing up the proportion of fruits and veggies in their diets is all the weight loss program they need. If that sounds suspiciously easy, just do a little arithmetic. Cutting out two soft drinks per day is about 240 calories. Cutting out a sweetened coffee can be even more. And a 300 calorie per day deficit is all you need for gentle weight loss.

The bottom line is that the current scientific consensus says that weight loss is best achieved through a moderate, sustained calorie deficit and moderate, sustained exercise.[8] It may not be easy for everybody, but it really is about that simple for almost everyone. Keep it real, and take it slow.

---

[8] https://theness.com/neurologicablog/index.php/more-on-weight-loss/

Chapter 6

When Food Gets Scary

A Brief Word About Eating Disorders

I hope it's clear that I do not want to frighten you. But please let me share one of the most frightening conversations I ever had. When my daughter was about 13 years old her pediatrician told me that she had *anorexia nervosa* (usually just called anorexia). I had heard of it, of course, but didn't know that much about it. He told me that it is the most lethal mental illness there is, with an extremely high mortality rate. Let me tell you, *that* got my attention.

We spent the next few years working to defeat it. It was not easy. It can, however, be done.

Eating disorders are scary serious business. This isn't a book about treating or diagnosing eating disorders. But since my daughter survived one I have some thoughts, and can anticipate some of the most common questions. I also think it's important that people who have an eating disorder know that they're not alone, they're not broken, and they're not bad people. So how about a short chapter in question and answer format? You can skip it if you're sure that eating disorders are not part of your life. Then again, you may meet someone some day who has one, and you'll know better what to do and, just as importantly, what not to do.

Q: How do I know if I have an eating disorder?

A: You don't. Not unless a doctor tells you. Nobody should attempt to self-diagnose this or any other mental illness. I can, though, give you a few things that should get your attention. If any of the following are true about you, please consider making an appointment right away with a qualified medical doctor:

- Restricting my food intake is a way to gain control over my life.
- I sometimes experience anxiety or dread when I sit down to a meal.
- There are "fear foods" that make me anxious.
- I hide the way I eat from my family and friends.
- Eating around other people makes me uncomfortable.
- If I wear baggy clothes nobody will notice that I'm losing weight.
- I'm a bad person and I need to be perfect.
- I can eat 500 calories per day and be perfectly fine.
- I drink a lot of water or tea right before meal time.
- Pro-Ana web sites give me a sense of community and support.
- I think a lot about extra things I can do to lose weight, such as cold baths and eating celery.

Any one of the above should have you making an appointment. If more than two or three are true, make the appointment *right now*. As in put down this book and pick up the phone. Remember that you cannot diagnose or treat your own eating disorder, and you cannot diagnose one in anybody else. Please don't try.

Q: What do I do if I'm afraid that my child has an eating disorder?

A: Say nothing to your child, and contact their doctor immediately. The checklist above applies here as well. If you see any of those behaviors, or notice that your child is losing weight *at all*, contact the doctor. **Be prepared to listen.** A lot. Do not try to "help". Instead ask the doctor and other members of your child's medical team (because you'll have one) what you can do to be supportive.

One of the frustrating things about dealing with an eating disorder is that it's so counter-intuitive. Not only must you never remark in any way on your child's weight, **you mustn't remark on how they look**. That means no telling your daughter that she looks pretty. Is that hard? Boy, howdy. One of the hardest things ever, for me, at least. But it's doable.

Do not talk about food. Do not talk about eating disorders. Do not talk about calories. Do not talk about weight. For the first part of recovery the doctors may want to keep your child's weight a secret from them. Keep it secret.

Do whatever you can to keep their life normal. You may have to get tough when it comes to making doctor appointments and taking prescribed medications. The rest of the time just be loving, supportive, and listen like crazy. Your child will actually guide you as to when it's OK to bring up different subjects. Be aware that eating disorders are frequently comorbid with depression. Watch for signs such as difficulty getting out of bed for school, withdrawing from friends, and self harm (such as cutting). Be prepared for psychotherapy, counseling, and/or medication. Be supportive. Did I mention that listening is important?

Late in her recovery my daughter and I vacationed in Italy. We were dining *al fresco* in Florence one night when she took a bite and I saw her face suddenly illuminate with amazement. "Dad—I understand now why you love food so much." I nearly floated out of my chair. That moment, when it comes, will be one of the happiest in your life. Hang in there until it does.

Q: How can I help my friend (or sibling) who has an eating disorder?

A: Don't. That is, don't try to help directly with the disorder. Don't give any advice. All the cautions I gave to parents above, namely not talking about food, disorders, etc. apply. That includes mentioning how they look or how much they weigh.

What you *can* do is be a friend. One of the most pernicious things about an eating disorder is that it not only robs the sufferer of the ability to see themselves correctly, but it tries to take over their life. The more normal you can keep their life, the more socially connected they remain, the greater their chance of recovery. Like I told their parents, do a lot of really careful listening. Just the feeling that they are being heard is of tremendous value. As recovery progresses, *they* will tell *you* what's OK to talk about. Let them set the limits.

If they go out to eat with you and perhaps other friends, that's a total win even if all they do is cut their salad into tiny bits and push it around their plate with a fork. Don't comment on it. Just enjoy their company and let them enjoy yours. Getting comfortable with eating around other people is no trifling matter for them. Just being out with friends is a big deal.

One of the things that made recovery so difficult for my daughter was people "helpfully" criticizing the foods she was eating. Orthorexic attitudes of, "that food is bad for you" or "don't eat that!" are extremely damaging. For most people having lots of sweet, fatty foods in their diet is a bad idea. For a recovering anorexic those foods are literally life saving. That's a big part of why I come down so hard on orthorexia in this book. As I say elsewhere, what or how much another person eats is none of your business unless you are their doctor. Please don't make life harder for someone in recovery.

Recovery is hard. Wicked hard. Anybody who recovers from an eating disorder is a total badass in my book. Treat them with the love and respect a total badass deserves. They'll thank you when they're able. It might take a while. Be patient.

A few years ago my daughter and I built a web site and produced a few short podcast episodes aimed specifically at families with eating disorders. We tried to demystify, destygmatize, and provide practical tips. We have yummy, high-density recipes that can be used during anorexia recovery, as well as links to resources. You may find it useful. Just go to RecoveryDad.com[1].

Q: Aren't anorexics lucky that they can stay so thin?

A: No. And anybody who would say that needs to see a doctor. Seriously. It was shocking and sickening how much of this my daughter had to face. You wouldn't *dream* of telling a cancer patient they were "lucky to be so thin", yet a horrifying number of people (sadly, mostly women) think that this kind of remark is OK. (Even more sadly, I know of people on chemo who *did* hear this. I find that horrifying, and I hope you do as well.) Anorexia, and other eating disorders, are serious mental illnesses. They are the most deadly mental illnesses. Someone who has one is literally in the process of dying. It is not a lifestyle choice. It is absolutely not a weight loss strategy. There is nothing remotely lucky about having one.

---

[1] www.recoverydad.com

I remember my daughter's nutritionist telling her that people would keep calling her pretty — right up to her first heart attack. Now, since you exhibited excellent discernment in buying this book I know that *you* aren't one of those who would say something so hurtful. But if you overhear anybody else saying something this offensive, slap them down (firmly but metaphorically) and don't let them get away with it. In part it's a symptom of that orthorexia in our society that correlates being thin with being good. I don't know that it's actually possible to be too rich, but I know for certain that you can be too thin.

Chapter 7

Beware Bad Advice

Nutritional BS Detector Kit

As we perambulate the grocery store and the internet we are constantly assaulted with misinformation. Use this brief Nutritional BS Detector to help filter out sources of bad information.

1. Anybody trying to scare you away from a food or an ingredient is probably selling something — and likely making stuff up. And they're almost certainly wrong.
2. Anybody claiming that they have the One True Diet is definitely making stuff up.
3. Anybody claiming that something is a superfood doesn't know what they're talking about. There are no superfoods. There are just foods.
4. Ignore people who use words like "detox", "toxins", "boost", "promotes", or "supports" in a nutritional or medical context.
5. If someone wants you to eat or drink a different way in order to change your body's pH or alkalinity, run the other way. That advice is not just stupid, but potentially dangerous.
6. If a diet has a name it's probably bogus.
7. Someone making claims for their pet theory/diet/supplement/superfood is probably wrong in direct proportion to how sure they are of themselves.
8. Words like "natural", "organic", "processed", "clean", and "GMO-free" are meaningless in a nutritional context. Mostly they're used in fear-based marketing.

9. If you are eating a healthy, varied diet then vitamins and other supplements are almost certainly a waste of money at best and a danger at worst. Of course, if your doctor has recommended a supplement to treat a diagnosed condition or deficiency, do take that supplement as directed. In general the entire supplement industry is not to be trusted.

10. Don't take medical or nutritional advice from anybody selling a product, such as a supplement. Even if they dress up like a doctor in their publicity photo.

11. Never take medical or nutritional advice from someone claiming to have special knowledge that "science" or "doctors" don't. Something like, "Health tips your doctor doesn't want you to know!" should send you screaming in the opposite direction.

12. Beware of doctors who also just happen to be selling something — books, supplements, salad dressings, fasting clinics, etc. Sadly, some high profile doctors are in the fear-for-profit business.

13. I have yet to encounter anything with the word *wellness* tacked on that didn't turn out to be flapdoodle.

Traditional Bad Information

There are a number of traditions which are mother lodes of bad medical and dietary advice. They are, at best, pre-scientific superstitions. Let's have a quick look at some of the bigger ones.

Homeopathy, which is literally the stupidest pseudoscience in the world. It was completely made up out of whole cloth two hundred years ago (before science based medicine existed), loosely based on vitalism, where "like cures like". Except that it takes the supposedly "active" ingredient and literally dilutes it in water (or sometimes alcohol) until not a single molecule of it remains. Not even one.

Many people think homeopathy means "natural" or "herbal". It doesn't. It literally just means water. Water which is supposed to magically retain a "memory" of the substances that used to be in it. By the time I drink it, I'd much rather that the water have completely forgotten about all the times it was fish pee. Or worse.

Traditional Chinese Medicine is not science based, and promotes some food-as-medicine ideas that are not only bad for people but very bad for the environment. The Vietnamese offshoot in particular has driven many rare species into extinction, all because of the supposed mythical powers of rare animal parts. There actually is no such thing as "Western medicine" or "Eastern medicine". Real medicine is science based, and everything else just isn't medicine.

Religion often provides dietary rules and restrictions. If you can eat a healthy diet, as defined in this book, and still be observant, then fine. But do not for a moment think that religious dietary rules are based in science. They're usually sourced in superstition and are more about fomenting obedience and group cohesion than anything else. If a religious rule clashes with science, go with the science.

Ayurveda has some of the craziest food myths I've ever encountered. If you see someone claiming that some food combination, such as egg and banana, is dangerous, or that certain foods should only be eaten at certain times of day, it's a safe bet that they got that information from Ayurveda. Believers claim that it is a science, and is "natural medicine".

The problem is that there is no such thing as "natural medicine". All medical modalities can be sorted into one of 3 buckets:

1. Science has shown that it works.
2. Science has shown that it doesn't work.
3. Science has not yet tested it.

Only #1 can be called medicine. The rest are not medicine. Homeopathy and acupuncture, for example, are in bucket #2. Pretty much all of Ayurveda is either in #2 or #3. The parts of it that can be called medicine are in #1, and there's no reason to call them Ayurvedic anymore.

As Dr. Harriet Hall puts it, Ayurveda is ancient superstition, not ancient wisdom.[1] Nobody should take health or diet advice from Ayurveda. Science is the best and only method we have to know what works.

Let's just pause here to point out that any food can be eaten along with any other food, at any time of day. If you like how they taste together, that's all you need to know about combining foods.

---

[1] https://www.csicop.org/specialarticles/show/ayurveda_ancient_superstition_not_ancient_wisdom

It's worth mentioning that pointing out the bogus nature of Ayurveda is not an insult to anybody nor their culture. Every culture has produced similar pre-scientific notions. It was Europe, for example, that gave us homeopathy and bloodletting.

Trendy Misinformation

I've already warned you to be on the lookout for fear-based marketing terms, such as organic, non-GMO, and natural. Beware also the idea of **clean food**. It has nothing to do with contaminants. It's just another orthorexic ploy to force a warped moral view onto various foods.[2] The term was coined by a Canadian fitness model named Tosca Reno, and it sure does sell books. The clean eating movement has proven particularly damaging to young women. Anna Cherry, writes:[3]

> Sometimes clean eating is vegan, sometimes it's raw vegan, sometimes it's omnivorous—but it's always touted as the wholesome, pure way to eat, regardless of its disciples' other food-related views. The face of clean eating is disproportionately young, attractive, female, white, and affluent enough to be able to regularly afford chia seeds, kale, and coconut sugar.

Did you notice the red flag words *wholesome*, and *pure*? A problem that she rightly points out is that this cliquish, obsessive view of food can be extremely damaging, and young women are particularly at risk. Cherry also correctly observes:

> When you start to view food through the lenses of morality, judgment, and restriction, you've got a recipe for disaster.

Plant biology professor Kevin Folta also notes that the very notion of "clean food" is an offensive marketing ploy.[4]

---

[2] https://nationalpost.com/life/food/the-new-religion-how-the-emphasis-on-clean-eating-has-created-a-moral-hierarchy-for-food

[3] https://www.healthyway.com/content/how-the-clean-eating-fad-is-taking-a-toll-on-young-women/

[4] https://medium.com/on-advertising/the-deeply-offensive-marketing-ploy-of-clean-food-ad983f135b4e

At a time when all of our affluent-world food is produced with tremendous care and regulation, and 21,000 people will die today from lack of nutrition, it is disgusting to see safe food demonized in a cheap marketing gimmick. When I sit down with any meal I am grateful for what I have. Every calorie represents tremendous time, labor, fuel, water, fertilizer, crop protection — safe, affordable, and abundant. This is why each morsel is prized and special to me. I always clean a plate, and usually someone else's.

Oversimplification

A lot of well-intentioned people, not just outright scammers, oversimplify. This is a natural human tendency. We want that simple answer, a handy heuristic, a cheat, a shortcut. Unfortunately that's rarely the right approach. Nature is messy. That's why science is hard. When you hear of someone promoting one thing as the cause for many ills, it's time to be skeptical. It's popular, for example, to claim that inflammation is a Bad Thing to be avoided. Eat the right magical diet, avoid inflammation, and presto! No more health problems. If only.[5]

Just the idea that there's such a thing as a "health food" or "junk food" is itself an oversimplification. The truth is that only diets, which are (or should be) complex can be healthy or unhealthy. Any food can be part of any kind of diet, including a healthy one.

Nobody is immune to the search for a magic bullet. Dr. Linus Pauling was a renowned chemist and physicist, a founder of both quantum chemistry and molecular biology. His scientific contributions are hard to exaggerate. And then something happened. We don't really know why, but he latched onto the idea that Vitamin C was the new Most Important Thing. He promoted megadoses of it as a treatment for a wide variety of diseases. But he was out of his field of expertise, and descended into defensive crankery late in life. All you'll get from big doses of Vitamin C is expensive pee.

Remember that it's easier to frighten people than to educate them. It's far easier to frighten them about a single thing than enlighten them about a nuanced, complicated set of things.

---

[5] https://skeptoid.com/episodes/4614

High Tech Hokum

The internet is a marvelous resource. Yet, as we now know all too well, it makes bad information just as easy to find as good information. So let's talk about how to spot credible web sites and weed out the nonsense. Again, there are no hard and fast rules. The following tips will have you being right far more often than you are wrong.

Does it have a store? This will weed out most conspiracy sites and cranks. If the site giving you health advice just *happens* to also sell supplements, food, books, or expensive clinical retreats (such as for long-term fasting) then you should be highly suspicious. A legitimate source of science will almost never have a shopping cart. (Except maybe to purchase scientific publications.)

Could it be run by a crank? If the site features a single doctor who appears in a photo wearing a white smock or scrubs (worse, with a stethoscope) your spidey senses should be tingling. By crank I mean someone who has gone rogue, setting themselves apart from the rest of science. Never trust a guru, or anybody claiming to be one. There is no one person with all the right answers in health or nutrition. People setting themselves up as gurus almost always lead you off into risky (and expensive) waters. This year there's even one claiming to be a "medical medium".[6] Yes, he "talks" to spirits and doles out medical advice about, strangely, the thyroid, which he has identified as the seat of all problems. (Talking to spirits is a piece of cake. Getting them to answer, on the other hand...) Typically these gurus promote a product, book, or diet that claims to have the One Right Answer to a lot of problems. *The more diseases that a thing is claimed to treat, the less you should believe the claims. Likewise, the more conditions blamed on a single organ or body system, the more likely it's all pseudoscience.*

Is it on this list? Brian Dunning is a well established skeptic and science communicator. If you haven't already, you should take a listen to his Skeptoid[7] podcast. He even has a channel dedicated to scientific food information, called The Feeding Tube. You can find it at feedingtube.tv.[8]

---

[6] https://sciencebasedmedicine.org/the-medical-mediums-thyroid-pseudoscience/
[7] https://skeptoid.com/
[8] https://feedingtube.tv/

In 2015 he published an updated list of the 10 worst anti-science web sites.[9] By this point it should not be a surprise that over half of them are dedicated all or in part to misinformation about food and health — and, of course, selling worthless products. So let me save you some time right now by giving you a head start on a list of known bogus web sites:

- Chopra.com
- FoodBabe.com
- DoctorOz.com
- InfoWars.com
- Mercola.com
- NaturalNews.com
- Whale.to

Some of those sources show up in an organic food industry confidential PR plan to spread fake science.[10] There may or may not be the name of a high-profile, best-selling author of books about food there as well.

This is as good a place as any to warn you off of **Naturopathy**. It is most certainly *not* medicine. Typically it's a license to sell worthless (or dangerous) supplements. They learn homeopathy in school. As Dr. Hall puts it, "What naturopaths do that is good is no different from what MDs do, and what they do that is different is not good, and is potentially dangerous."

The TV Doctors

There's a special category that overlaps with diet and just overall health advice, namely TV doctors. The prime example is Dr. Mehmet Oz. He's a sad and frustrating case because, by all reports, he's a highly competent surgeon. It's worth pointing out that while doctors *use* science most doctors don't *do* science, and surgeons even less. But the big danger seems to be when a fat TV contract is dangled in front of them. Some, and only some, of Dr. Oz's advice is common sense and reasonable. But far too much of it is dangerous quackery, something he does to sell products, not guard your health.

---

[9] https://skeptoid.com/episodes/4495
[10] https://geneticliteracyproject.org/2018/06/19/how-the-organic-industry-spreads-fake-science/

And he's not the only one. A prospective study published in the medical journal *BMJ* in 2015 took random samples of 40 episodes each of *The Dr. Oz Show* and *The Doctors*, and evaluated the medical advice given.[11] The results weren't great. Dr. Steven Novella, writing on *Science Based Medicine*, gives the summary:[12]

> They found that, for *The Dr. Oz Show*, there was some evidence to support the advice 46% of the time, the evidence contradicted the advice 15% of the time, and there was no evidence either way 39% of the time. *The Doctors* fared a little better, with 63%, 14%, and 24% respectively.

Ouch. Think about what a low bar "some evidence" is. So even when we give Dr. Oz points for being sorta right, he's still mostly wrong more than half the time. And about one out of seven times he's flat out wrong. So beware of doctors on TV, especially if they use words like *miracle*. There are no miracles in science, let alone in nutrition.

Doctors who want to be gurus, who have products or programs to sell, or who use any of the red flag terms in our BS Detector, should be approached with your skepticism cranked up to eleven.

Beware the magazine rack

We've all seen those magazines in the check-out aisle or the beauty salon. I'm not talking about the tabloids which you're already smart enough not to rely on for any kind of information, much less diet advice. I mean "health" and "women's" magazines. Most covers are a slaw of hokum and buzzwords. Just today I saw a magazine cover from a "women's magazine" (it even has *woman* in the title). This is a good, real-world opportunity to test your new BS Detector. Here are the stories being teased:

- New Research! The veggie that makes your brain 11 YEARS YOUNGER
- The fingertip trick that MAKES HAIR GROW

---

[11] https://www.bmj.com/content/349/bmj.g7346
[12] https://sciencebasedmedicine.org/tv-doctors-give-unreliable-recommendations/

- An herbal cure for TUMMY TROUBLE
- PROTECT YOUR HEART just by watching this on TV —40% reduction in risk!
- CRANKY *and* CREAKY? A common melon cures *both*!
- Discovered! The all-natural cure for FALL ALLERGIES

And the capper:

- Lose 25 pounds in 10 days on Dr. Oz's LIVER DETOX. Eating *more* fat helps your liver burn fat! "Your liver will get you skinny!"

There was also something about a dessert recipe, which is probably fine, and tips for saving money, which may or may not be so fine. You can see all the red flags, right? Every single thing on the list you just read is unadulterated flapdoodle and codswallop. Magazines like this are insulting at best and dangerous at worst. Dr. Oz's horrible advice to attempt losing 25 pounds in 10 days could really injure someone.

Magazines with slicker covers, selling fitness, yoga, organic, or whatever's trendy, can be just as deceptive, even if they do have better graphic design. Remember that their goal is really to sell magazines and give your eyeballs to advertisers, not to promote science or healthy eating.

This little guide will eliminate the vast majority of bogus, dishonest, or dangerous claims. As always, go with what your doctor says. If they sent you to a competent dietician or nutritionist, then follow that advice. Remember that this book is about general cases. A book that claims to know what is best for *you* is a great candidate for the recycling bin. Or maybe cutting up to make art projects, if you're the creative type.

Ransom notes, maybe.

Water woo

Let's talk water for a minute. As the most ubiquitous and necessary nutrient it has, expectedly, accumulated perhaps the greatest amount of nonsense. The myths around water go far beyond the old 8 glasses per day myth.

There are people, and traditions, which claim to tell you what temperature your water should be. They claim that it makes a difference, completely ignoring the fact that no matter what temperature it is in your glass (or mug) it's going to be at body temperature within seconds. If it isn't burning you, and still flows as a liquid, then it's fine. If you ingest ice, try to let it melt in your mouth before swallowing, so you don't choke on it. Neither water at various temperatures, nor foods, are "cooling" or "heating". They all just end up at body temperature, so enjoy food at the temperature you like.

A lot of charlatans sell wicked expensive machines to ionize and alkalize your water, which is supposed to provide another suspiciously long list of "health benefits". Since pure water isn't conductive, you have to add some kind of impurity to ionize. Naturally, the same charlatans will happily sell you a very expensive solution to add to the water. It's almost as expensive as the machine. And do you know what simple home solution you could add to the water to do exactly the same thing?

Bleach. Go ahead and ask your doctor if you should be supplementing bleach in your diet.

There are brands willing to do all of this nonsense to your water and bottle it for you. It's known as Kangen water[13]. They claim, well, a lot of crazy stuff. One way or another, if you want woo water you're going to have to cough up a lot of money for it.

Fortunately this is mostly just a waste of money, because if you ate or drank something that actually changed the pH of your blood very much then you'd probably get a ride in either an ambulance or a hearse.

Or you can drop big bucks to consume oxygenated water. Made properly, it really does have extra oxygen in it. But until someone figures out a way to breath through their digestive tract, there's no reason to expect oxygen in your water to do a lick of good. Just keep breathing. Your lungs are pretty good at getting oxygen right out of the air. For free!

There are traditions, mostly Ayurvedic, that tout all sorts of benefits from having some combination of lemon, garlic, or apple cider vinegar in your water. All any of that does, really, is change the flavor of the water. There's nothing wrong with flavoring your water — just ask an herbal

---

[13] https://sciencebasedmedicine.org/down-the-virtual-rabbit-hole/

tea drinker. But don't expect any magical "health benefits". In fact, by now, it should be pretty clear that the term "health benefits" on anything should be seen as a red flag, not a selling point.

Ayurveda even recommends drinking gold, silver, or copper water. That's something which doesn't actually exist.[14] Those metals don't even dissolve in water. It's like homeopathy, but even more stupid because there's no active ingredient to dilute into nothingness.

But the water fad that really takes the cake is "raw water". This fad caught on recently in Silicon Valley, and is almost the *ad absurdum* of the appeal to nature. The idea — get this — is to bottle completely untreated water: bacteria, amoebas, dirt, and all, and sell it to gullible rich people because it's *natural*.[15] Well, it sure as shooting *is* natural. But remember that most of nature has nothing better to do than try to kill you. Proponents even tried to say that seeing it turn green in the bottle was a feature, not a bug. Hey, it's probiotic![16] I kid you not. As it turns out, there are very many good reasons why we purify our drinking water supply. Among those reasons are bacteria, amoebas, and dirt.

There's so much bad information out there about water that I'll bet an entire web site could be dedicated to just water hoaxes.

Oh, look! Here's just such a web site: It's www.chem1.com/CQ[17] —also known as H2O.con. (Con, not com. See what they did there? C'mon. Let the scientist be funny.)

The 30-Second Detox

All the detox you need!

Yes, folks, here it is! You want to get toxins out of your body? Here's how, and it takes only seconds:

Pee. And keep breathing.

Your liver and kidneys provide all the detox you'll ever need, assuming that you don't actually get poisoned. In the latter case the hospital

---

[14] https://www.skepdoc.info/gold-water-silver-water-copper-water/
[15] https://sciencebasedmedicine.org/raw-water-latest-dangerous-natural-health-fad/
[16] https://www.snopes.com/fact-check/raw-water-provide-probiotic-health-benefits/
[17] http://www.chem1.com/CQ/

may use some more advanced treatments. The point is that every single "detox" claim on the market is utter codswallop. As Neil DeGrasse Tyson put it, "The likelihood that a person uses the word 'toxin' correlates strongly with how much chemistry the person does *not* know." That's why talking about "toxins" is a huge red flag that should steer you clear of the rest of that person's advice.

Modern life has not filled you with dangerous toxins. You do not get toxins out of your body through perspiration. There is no toxin crisis. There are no toxins building up on your intestinal or colonic walls. You don't get a detox from juice, from an enema, or from fasting.

By now the pattern should be familiar: Frighten you about something and then offer to sell you the cure. Toxins sound bad! Ooh, toxins! Please help me rid my body of toxins!

Yeah, well, your internal organs already do a bang up job at that. You don't need any special foods, elixirs, or exercises to do better. Just remember to pee. And don't postpone it too long, lest you suffer the ignominious fate of Tycho Brahe. In a superhuman effort to be polite to his hostess at a party he delayed going to the Little Astronomer's room far too long and died from a ruptured bladder. That's a totally avoidable tragedy.

The only supplement you need is a chill pill

Vitamin supplements are almost always a ripoff.

If you're eating a variety of foods, mostly plants, with plenty of veggies and fruits, you almost certainly get enough vitamins and other micronutrients (such as minerals). There is no need for you to take a vitamin or other supplement unless your medical doctor has recommended one to treat a diagnosed deficiency or condition.

That's worth repeating: Don't take *any* vitamins or supplements unless the doctor says to. I know that sounds strange after decades of highly effective advertising and propaganda that even equates giving vitamin pills to children as a sign of motherly love. But it's true.

Note that if you are a vegan you'll have to be extra conscientious about vitamins and may need to supplement your B vitamins, especially B-12. This is part of why the current scientific consensus is that diets that include *some* meat yield the best results. Personally I don't think a diet that requires supplementation can be considered a complete diet, but it's clearly possible to live a healthy life as a vegan as long as you make sure you get the vitamins you need and eat a big variety. After all, a diet of just french fries and Oreo cookies would be vegan. It would also be unhealthily narrow.

Do not risk a vitamin B-12 deficiency. The effects are both dire and permanent. For a saucy deep-dive into the subject see the Angry Chef's blog post series, *Diets in a Time of Scurvy*[18].

The rest of us, though, are beset by a supplement industry that is an under-regulated, greedy monster. Note again that pretty much every pitch they make to you is one of fear: Take this supplement or you won't feel healthy, won't live long, might get a horrible disease. In America we literally flush billions of dollars a year down the toilet, all thanks to the supplement industry.

Your body doesn't need big doses of any vitamins or minerals. That's why they're called *micro*nutrients. If you get more than you need of some vitamins, such as Vitamin C, it just gets flushed out through the kidneys. That's why some say that Americans have the most expensive pee in the world. But some vitamins can accumulate. It's possible to overdose on some vitamins, such as A and E.

As with anything else, *more is not better*. Just like getting too many antioxidants is bad for you, getting too much of some vitamins will do you harm.

Wait. You didn't know that about antioxidants? Yup. Your body needs and uses some, but getting too many can even be harmful.[19] Eat your fruits and veggies. Never buy antioxidant supplements. Realizing that too much isn't good for you, and looking at the absurd quantities on vitamin labels will make it clear why not.[20]

Multivitamins are almost never a good idea. It would take a rare case for a doctor to recommend them, because they contain wildly varying amounts of various vitamins. If you have an actual deficiency then a

---

[18] https://angry-chef.com/blog/diets-in-a-time-of-scurvy-part-1/
[19] https://sciencebasedmedicine.org/more-trouble-for-antioxidants/
[20] https://sciencebasedmedicine.org/a-call-for-caution-on-antioxidant-supplementation/

supplement with that specific, targeted vitamin is far more likely to be helpful. If your doctor doesn't tell you to take a multivitamin, all it's doing is lightening your bank account and making your urine expensive.

You are almost assuredly not deficient in Vitamin D. If you've heard the notion that you lack Vitamin D and really need to supplement it, it's likely the work of Dr. Michael Holick. His work has been funded primarily by — are you sitting down? — The manufacturers of Vitamin D supplements and the labs that do Vitamin D tests.[21] Oh, and tanning salons. There's no evidence that people with high Vitamin D levels are any healthier than those with lower levels. There is no reason to even screen for your Vitamin D levels if you are asymptomatic. In other words, if your doctor doesn't think you need a Vitamin D test, don't bother.[22]

Do you need Vitamin D? Yup, it's a vital hormone. But if you eat a decent diet and get a little sun now and then the odds are that your Vitamin D levels are just dandy. Vitamin D will not prevent the flu, and is not a substitute for the flu shot you should be getting every season.

The bottom line is that routine vitamin supplementation is mostly useless[23]. And, no, it doesn't even help with vascular disease.[24] See? I've saved you even more money.

Beware of fake vitamins. There are cranks who insist that cancer is caused by a deficiency in Vitamin B17, and who will happily sell you doses of the stuff. The first problem is that there is no such thing as Vitamin B17. That's just a name slapped on a bogus drug called *laetrile* in an effort to skirt around regulations. Its inventor was a crank named Dr. Ernst Krebs[25] who, working alone in San Francisco in the 1920's, dreamed up the idea that an extract from apricot pits could reduce tumors in rats. The resulting drug, laetrile, was later thoroughly tested and the result was that it did nothing to treat cancer, but was potentially highly toxic. So, yes, under the guise of sounding "natural" there are people willing to sell you a useless poison.

[21] https://www.nytimes.com/2018/08/18/business/vitamin-d-michael-holick.html
[22] https://sciencebasedmedicine.org/vitamin-d-to-screen-or-not-to-screen/
[23] https://sciencebasedmedicine.org/routine-vitamin-supplementation-mostly-useless/
[24] https://sciencebasedmedicine.org/multivitamins-and-vascular-disease/
[25] https://www.snopes.com/fact-check/cancer-vitamin-b17-deficiency/

And that's just vitamins. The rest of the supplement industry is even worse.

I could probably fill a whole chapter with the risks of "harmless-sounding" supplements, but my goal is to educate, not frighten you. To vaccinate your mind against the supplement and "wellness" industry, though, consider the case of a man who took green tea extract in the hopes of avoiding an early death due to heart disease, as happened to his father, and ended up damaging his liver.[26] In fact, so many crazy claims are made for green tea that we're going to take a detour to talk about just that.

You can read about it in more depth on Science Based Medicine[27], but the gist is:

- It's maybe effective at reducing some health risks.
- It's not recommended for any conditions.
- It can increase many health risks, especially liver problems. It may even interfere with some cancer treatments. (Even when consumed as tea and not an extract.)

The section on safety says:

> The Natural Medicines Comprehensive Database gives green tea a rating of **"likely safe"** when used as a beverage in moderate amounts, as **"possibly safe"** when used as an extract for up to 6 months, as **"possibly unsafe"** for long-term use in high doses due to its caffeine content, and as **"likely unsafe"** when used orally in very high doses. It reports a long list of adverse reactions including liver failure. It reports a long list of interactions with other supplements and with drugs, and warns that green tea may worsen symptoms of various diseases.

In the end it's just tea. Have a little if you enjoy the taste. Don't overdo it, and don't expect magic to happen. What, even, is a dietary supplement? It's not really a scientific term, but a regulatory one. The FDA definition[28] reads:

---

[26] https://theness.com/neurologicablog/index.php/liver-failure-from-green-tea-extract/

[27] https://sciencebasedmedicine.org/green-tea-panacea-or-poison/

[28] https://www.fda.gov/food/dietary-supplements

> A dietary supplement is a product intended for ingestion that contains a "dietary ingredient" intended to add further nutritional value to (supplement) the diet.

Vague enough for you? Not vague enough for the supplement industry. That definition might actually be alright if that's what they stuck to. Unfortunately for those of us in the U.S., the supplement industry has two powerful senators in its fish-oil-lined pockets, especially Orrin Hatch,[29] the senator from Utah, the headquarter state of the supplement racket. He and Tom Harkin, a fan of pseudoscience in general, gave us the anti-consumer monstrosity known as the DSHEA, or Dietary Supplement Health and Education Act[30] of 1994. There they weaseled in "herbs and botanicals" to the list of supplements.

It's essentially a gigantic loophole which allows selling ineffective, potentially dangerous flapdoodle with a science-sounding halo on it. While they aren't technically allowed to claim that their un-tested products have actual medical effects, they're allowed to use deceptive language such as "supports bladder health" or "boosts metabolism". When you see "supports" or "boosts" in any product claim, just put it back on the shelf and keep walking.

Speaking of fish oil, you may or may not be surprised to learn that there are no particular gains from taking those expensive fish oil capsules. A meta analysis showed no clear health benefit to supplementing Omega-3.[31] In fact, Paul Greenberg wrote a whole book, *The Omega Principle*,[32] on both the paucity of scientific backing for supplementation, but the potentially severe environmental impact of producing fish oil tablets.

Herbs and botanicals are not taken to "add further nutritional value to the diet" no matter what the FDA was legally forced to say. You can prove that yourself by looking at the ads for any of them: They're really pitched as drugs.

---

[29] https://sciencebasedmedicine.org/utahs-senator-orrin-hatch-defender-of-the-supplement-industry/

[30] https://sciencebasedmedicine.org/dshea-a-travesty-of-a-mockery-of-a-sham/

[31] https://sciencebasedmedicine.org/no-benefit-from-fish-oil/

[32] https://slate.com/technology/2018/08/omega-3s-are-useless-for-you-and-terrible-for-the-environment.html

Due to the Brobdingnagian loophole created by the DSHEA, scammers (by which I mean the supplement industry) are selling dangerous nonsense to treat diseases.

Now I'm going to give you a secret that THEY don't want you to know.

(And by THEY I mean the scammers.) It's *technically* illegal for them to sell herbs and botanicals as medicine. And they have *technically* covered their leather-cradled asses by including a tiny bit of boilerplate on their products. This bit of text is known as the Quack Miranda Warning:

> **This / these statement(s) have not been evaluated by the Food and Drug Administration. This product is not intended to diagnose, treat, cure or prevent any disease.**

Now, I know you're already thinking that this book has paid for itself by letting you skip the organic surcharge at the supermarket, and stop subscribing to vitamins on Amazon. But it doesn't stop there, oh no! Whenever you see the Quack Miranda Warning from now on, you will know that it really means:

> **This product is a potentially dangerous ripoff. Do not buy it.**

As usual, the only exception is if your medical doctor has recommended the supplement to treat a specific, diagnosed condition. In that case a good doctor will usually have a recommendation as to a specific brand and product. Why? Because supplements are still worse than you think.

Supplements can poison you.

Since the DSHEA lets the industry set its own standards (what could go wrong?) its standards are, shockingly, often rather low. **When you buy a supplement you are getting an unknown dose of an untested ingredient of unknown purity and with unknown amounts of contaminants.** In other words, you have no idea what you just bought. A

2017 study[33] tabulated the "out-of-hospital dietary supplement exposures reported to the National Poison Data System from 2000 through 2012" and found:

> There were 274,998 dietary supplement exposures from 2000 through 2012. The annual rate of dietary supplement exposures per 100,000 population increased by 46.1% during 2000–2002, decreased 8.8% during 2002–2005, and then increased again by 49.3% from 2005 to 2012. These trends were influenced by the decrease in ma huang exposures starting in 2002.

Interestingly, the rise in toxic events[34] paused briefly in 2003 when the FDA banned *ma huang*. This is apparently the only time the FDA managed to get an herbal supplement off the market in the lifetime of the DSHEA.

Even if a specific herb were shown scientifically to have a medical benefit, there's no way to know if you're actually getting it. You may buy a bottle with Gingko on the label, but really get alfalfa and rice flour. I've already warned you about both TCM (Traditional Chinese Medicine) and weight loss supplements. Besides not working for weight loss, you can get this sort of thing:[35]

> In Belgium in the early 1990s, the TCM herb Stephania tetrandra was used for weight loss. Aristolochia fangchi was mistakenly used instead, and this resulted in more than 100 cases of renal failure and more than 20 cases of urothelial dysplasia. Similar problems were later reported in the UK. The culprit is thought to be the aristolochic acid found in Aristolochia fangchi. In TCM practice, Stephania tetrandra and Aristolochia fangchi were never meant to be used for weight loss.

If you start with superstition and add snake oil, bad things are going to happen. The industry is so cavalier about its customers that you literally don't know what you're getting when you buy most supplements, no matter how many times they use marketing jargon like "pure" and "natural"

---

[33] https://link.springer.com/article/10.1007/s13181-017-0623-7

[34] https://sciencebasedmedicine.org/increase-in-supplement-poisonings/

[35] https://www.ncbi.nlm.nih.gov/pmc/articles/PMC2700222/

on the label. The FDA looked at hundreds and found them contaminated by prescription drugs, often more than one.[36]

This is just the tip of the iceberg. Supplements are, at best, a waste of money. At worst they can hurt you very badly. Skip them unless the doctor says otherwise. You're healthier and richer for it.

Fortunately, writes Dr. Novella,[37] it seems that the tide is starting to turn. A recent Business Insider article essentially lays out the "supplement con" and...

> ...challenges the major narrative promoted by the supplement industry – that supplements are safe, effective, natural, and actually in the bottle. If we are lucky, this may mark the start of a sea change in how Americans see supplements.

Herbal poisons

A lot of herbal supplements straight up carry the risk of poisoning you. Kratom, an Asian herb currently trending, has opioid effects, can be lethal at high doses, and really should be considered a serious drug. Right now it's unregulated and sold as a supplement. Some so-called homeopathic teething products turned out not to be homeopathic at all (because actual homeopathy is just water), but contained toxic doses of belladonna.[38] Not what you want to be giving to your baby, no matter how fussy.

The word "herbal" has taken on that same halo as "natural", and it can't be trusted either. Herbs can contain significant doses of who-knows-what, and are often sold in unknown strengths with unknown contaminants. Just because something is "herbal" doesn't make it safe, let alone healthy.

---

[36] https://www.scientificamerican.com/article/hundreds-of-dietary-supplements-are-tainted-with-prescription-drugs/

[37] https://sciencebasedmedicine.org/the-supplement-con/

[38] https://sciencebasedmedicine.org/fda-warns-about-homeopathic-teething-products/

Pregnancy

One of those diagnosed conditions that requires vitamins is pregnancy. There is no evidence that expecting mothers should take multivitamins and iron, but the science is clear that they should supplement Vitamin B9, or folic acid. In fact, women who might become pregnant should take it, because the birth defects it prevents can happen early.[39] Your doctor will surely tell you. Believe them.

Don't confuse food with medicine

> "Let food be thy medicine and
> medicine be thy food."
> — Attributed to Hypocrites

That sage advice is pretty good, except for one thing: It's wrong. Of course there are diseases and conditions that can be treated by diet. Malnutrition and scurvy are obvious examples. That doesn't make food medicinal. It just means that a healthy diet can correct for deficiencies and, to some extent, lower your odds of some diseases.

The trouble comes when nature-worshipping orthorexics get the notion that they can skip actual medicine, and even avoid seeing the doctor when ill, as long as they eat the right magical foods. I already mentioned how we probably lost Steve Jobs too soon because he tried to treat cancer with a vegan diet rather than the surgery and medical treatments that were indicated.

It's a sign of an obsessive, unhealthy relationship to food when you choose what to eat based on what sort of medicinal value it's supposed to have. Don't mistake food for medicine.

---

[39] https://sciencebasedmedicine.org/prenatal-multivitamins-and-iron-not-evidence-based/

Chapter 8

The Joy of Food

How to Eat

If you're a typical American you know that your diet probably needs a little help. Maybe a lot. For any changes to be meaningful, they have to be long term. And by long term I mean for the rest of your life. Sound daunting? It turns out that there are some very simple steps you can take which have been scientifically demonstrated to make significant improvements to how you eat.

Eat your veggies first.

Oh, that sounds too simple, doesn't it? It works. At home, serve and eat the vegetable course first, before bringing out any of the other food. That can be the salad, the spuds, whatever. As long as it's vegetables. This one step works to tune your diet toward the proportion it should have. You don't have to do anything special beyond that in order to get the benefit. After a while you just may decide to up the plant part of your diet even more, which would be dandy. For now, just eat your veggies first.

Use small barriers.

Picture yourself seated at a table, say reading a book. Shouldn't be a big stretch. There's a small bowl of candy right by your fingertips. Imagine how much candy you'll eat. Now conjure the same situation, but with the candy bowl at the opposite end of the table. Experiments have shown quite consistently that you'll eat a lot less candy that way. Surprised? Psychology is weird, but it works.

If a barrier that small is effective, imagine not having the candy in the house at all. I hasten to point out that there's nothing wrong with candy. If you like candy then you should have some. *Some.* Since it should obviously form a small part of your healthy diet, make it an every now and then treat. If candy is your kryptonite, *don't keep any in the house.* Whatever it is that you know you should eat less of, just don't buy it at the grocery store. Instead perhaps save it for special visits to places such as bakeries, ice cream shops, and even candy stores.

Watch the added sugar.

A simple way to get your sugar intake under control is to cut way down on sugary drinks. That means sugary soda pop, loaded up coffee drinks, milk shakes, and fruit juice. Yes, fruit juice. Nutritionally it's nearly identical to soda pop: It's water, sugar, and some flavor. It may also have some vitamins. Big whoop.

That doesn't mean you can't ever have a sugary drink. Like any other food, as long as it's in proper proportion it's not a problem. Note, though, that a single serving of pop or juice can shoot your entire day's added sugar allowance. If you've been in the habit of drinking a juice and sweetened coffee in the morning and a couple of pops during the day, you can see where that leaves you. It's good to be sweet, but not that sweet.

You could try what I did, and switch mostly to water. It only took a couple of weeks and I found I preferred it. But you could also switch to beverages with non-nutritive, or low-calorie sweeteners. Those are sometimes, somewhat incorrectly, called artificial sweeteners. What they really are are substances that taste sweet (making them real sweeteners) but don't give you any calories. Or at least too few to bother counting. But you've heard scary things about them, right? Remember what we said about people trying to frighten you? It applies here as well. As long as you don't have the very rare genetic disorder that requires you to steer clear of Aspartame,[1] you have nothing to worry about with non-nutritive

---

[1] https://sciencebasedmedicine.org/are-artificial-sweeteners-safe/

sweeteners in anything even remotely resembling the amount you'd get in a reasonable diet. The latest science[2] still shows them to be safe, and a valid part of weight control:[3]

> Low-calorie sweeteners provide a means to reduce energy density while largely preserving food or beverage reward value. Consistent with this, consumption of low-calorie sweeteners compared with consumption of sugars has been found to reduce energy intake and body weight.

For many people, just cutting sweet drinks is enough to completely manage their sugar intake and even their weight. It's worth a try. If you're currently habituated to having sweet beverages every day, or multiple times per day, try just stopping. It may be hard at first, but after about a week or two of drinking mostly water you'll find that you don't miss it much. You can, of course, have a sweet drink (like a shake, or that expensive coffee, or even a soda pop) every now and then. Want a couple of sugars in your coffee? No problem. You're just likely to have an easier time eating a healthy diet if you make them occasional treats rather than a habit.

While you're being smart about hydration, remember that water is just water. See *Water Woo* in the chapter *Beware Bad Advice* for more.

Eat when you're hungry.

Just as there is no One True Diet, there is no One True Meal Schedule. If you're comfortable and functioning well, the number of meals you have in a day, and what hours you eat them, are entirely arbitrary. That doesn't keep lots of people, including wannabe gurus, from extolling the virtues of this, that, or the other eating schedule.

You may have heard that breakfast is the most important meal of the day, or that eating close to bed time will cause weight gain. The problem with the former is that breakfast is merely the first meal you eat each day, not the time of day you eat it nor the kind of food you eat. No meal is more important than another. The problem with the latter is that it's just a myth.

---

[2] https://sciencebasedmedicine.org/update-on-low-calorie-sweeteners/
[3] https://www.ncbi.nlm.nih.gov/pubmed/30290075

Having said that, there are nuances. People who have trouble sleeping are recommended to keep to a regular eating schedule. It doesn't matter much what it is, as long as it's the same every day. Also, going to bed hungry can lower your sleep quality. It's possible for hunger cues to arouse the brain enough to interrupt good sleep, yet not wake you all the way up. If you want a bedtime snack, favor high-satiety foods that are predominantly proteins and fats, and downplay quick-digesting foods high in carbs and sugars. Nuts and eggs are better for this job than cookies or crackers, for example.

You don't need three meals per day. That schedule was really the result of industrialization, and was most convenient for factory workers. If you'd rather have one, two, four, or five meals per day it doesn't really make a difference. For that matter, you can't even precisely define a "meal". When does a snack become a meal? When you eat sitting at a table? One limit is that many dentists recommend not splitting your day into more than six meals. That has more to do with oral hygiene than nutrition.

Be wary of any argument on meal times that appeals to evolution. The phrase "we evolved to…" is very frequently followed by pure fantasy. For most of our species' history there were no meal schedules at all. We ate when we could, and went hungry when we couldn't. If you are in a position to choose when you eat, you're free to choose. Evolution won't judge you.

There's a fad called intermittent fasting, which is very ill-defined. The term is a little nonsensical, because unless you eat while you sleep you're fasting intermittently every day. In normal usage it can mean anything from just having a late breakfast to going days without food. Late breakfast is fine, starving for days not so much. The most sensible version claims that you should get all of your calories within an eight-hour block of the day. I'd call that an "extended daily fast" rather than intermittent fasting.

There is some preliminary evidence of positive benefits for an extended daily fast.[4] And by preliminary I do mean preliminary. One study was encouraging enough to be able to claim that more studies are needed.

---

[4]http://stm.sciencemag.org/content/9/377/eaai8700

If you're comfortable going at least 16 hours between meals, then by all means do this version of "intermittent fasting". It won't hurt. If not, don't worry about it. Eat on whatever schedule keeps you happy, functioning, at a stable weight, and healthy. You do not have to conform to anybody else's schedule.

Drink when you're thirsty. Drink mostly water, and go easy on the sugary drinks. We already talked about why.

Try Something New

Since I'm plugging variety, it makes sense to try lots of new foods when you can. It's not only healthy, but fun. Of course you have some favorites already, most of them being what you grew up with. It turns out that your food preferences are almost completely habitual. Your genetics have little to nothing to do with it. Exceptions are things like some people born with the curse of having cilantro taste like soap. But that's rare. For just about any food, you like what you eat for long enough.

This is known as habituation. When you were an infant your mom wasn't giving you options, so you learned to like what you got. Naturally your own favorites emerged over time. But there is pretty much no food that you cannot learn to like. You will habituate to anything you eat regularly for six to eight weeks. The kicker, as I'll explain again later, is that you don't have to eat much of it. In fact, a serving the size of a single pea will work. This technique is called microbites, and it's so cool that I'll remind you of it again in the next section when we talk about children and food.

So as you learn to cook, and go exploring in your supermarket's produce aisle, try something new now and then. And if you think you'd like to like it, just keep eating it for a while.

Helping Children Love Food

The best time to forge a healthy relationship with food is when we are little. Parents, especially new ones, are understandably concerned about their child's nutrition. Unfortunately the desire to be a good parent can, if taken to an extreme, make one not such a good parent. This would be a good time to go watch *Finding Nemo* in case you need a reminder of the risks of over-parenting. Fear mongers know that parents of babies are easy prey. The concern, the stress, and the love can all make us susceptible to fear-based messages that aren't good for us — or for our children.

Some of the best advice parents can get is *relax*. Hey. I should work that word into the title of a book. Don't let stress have any part of meal time. Don't fret that little Sweet Pea didn't eat all of their carrots. Food should be fun and enjoyable. And messy. Don't forget how much fun messy food can be. For adults as well. A favorite Mexican saying is, "If you don't make a mess, you don't know how to eat mango."

Let's start with baby's arrival. Once that groovy extension cord connected to mom gets cut, it's a lifetime of oral alimentation ahead. Mom, if you can and want to breast feed, then that's awesome. Breast milk evolved to be just about the ideal food for your little poop machine. But it's not required. Under no circumstances let anybody berate you or make you feel diminished if you want or need to feed the baby with formula. There is absolutely nothing wrong with formula. You are not a bad mom if you feed your kid formula. You might be a bad mom if you don't feed your kid at all, though, and some moms have been so shamed by the Boob Mafia that they let their kid go a little hungry rather than supplement with formula. Posh. Let baby eat until satisfied, and give them an extra snuggle.

Oh, and under no circumstances give your nursing infant (under 6 months old) water. Breast milk and/or formula is fine. Water is not. It can interfere with the absorption of nutrients by making baby feel full, or even cause a deadly electrolyte imbalance known as water intoxication. Once baby is a little older then occasional sips are okay.

And now baby is sitting up happily in the high chair, massaging, throwing, mixing, painting with, and occasionally eating solid food. Sweet! This is a great opportunity to get in the habit of a wide variety. At this age they will try just about anything anyway. (Just *try* to keep random things out of their mouth. Hah! That's a big part of how they explore the world.)

As toddlers children start learning what foods they'll like. This is an even better time to try a variety. But go easy on the kid: It's quite normal to develop some favorites at this age and then go on to enjoy other foods later. Remember that at this stage their sense of taste is highly sensitive, so flavors that you enjoy as an adult might overwhelm them. Be patient.

Did you know that your food preferences are essentially all acquired? It's not like people from India have genes for Indian food while Swedish parents pass on Swedish food genes. With very rare exceptions there is almost no genetic or heritable component to food preferences. It turns out that we like —wait for it— what we eat as children. It's all a matter of habituation.

Remember what I was saying earlier about habituation and micro-bites? Kids can learn to like pretty much *anything* that they eat regularly for 6–8 weeks. This is why there's never anything quite like what your mom cooked for you: She cooked it for you a lot.

A pea-sized serving of a new food is pretty easy to turn into a fun game for a toddler, so you can habituate them to just about anything with a little patience. A toddler can even learn to like Brussels Sprouts. Honest. It's been done.

So your child is now sitting at their own chair, fully verbal and with many opinions about many things. It's not too late to expand their palate with habituation. But it's also not too early to seriously damage their relationship with food, even accidentally.

There are so many unhealthy notions about food which get fed to kids starting at an early age. In much of the world it's worse for girls than boys, but everybody gets hit with them. Do what you can to prepare your kids for the onslaught, and for goodness sake don't add to it. All of the things you're learning in this book about how to identify and avoid fear-based food messages will help. Mostly you just want to model a healthy relationship with food.

Don't forget to invite them to prepare food with you. Cooking is a vital life skill, and there's nothing quite as fun as the bonding you can do with your kids in the kitchen. Teach them the right way to use the tools and let them experiment as long as they can be safe.

And now, a vital message.

Never tell them they are fat. Never tell them they are skinny. In fact, you should never mention your child's weight to them. Ever. At all. I mean it. If you are concerned about their weight, talk to their doctor and let the doctor talk to them about it, if appropriate. Should they need to lose some weight the doctor will likely just have you adjust their diet a little. The child doesn't need to be told. You should be eating that healthy diet along with them anyway. You know: a variety of foods, mostly plants, with plenty of vegetables and fruits, not too much and not too little. Too many eating disorders have their roots in kids being told they're fat. It's incredibly damaging.

You'll have to prepare them, unfortunately, for other people commenting on their weight. There are even schools that think it's their business to weigh your children. Their intentions may be good, but it's an outrage, and can be incredibly damaging. (Let's just say that there's a high school PE teacher out there who had better hope we never meet in person.) You have my permission to let your school know that what your child weighs is none of their business, because it isn't. Sadly, it's probably going to happen anyway. At least your children will know better than to comment on anybody else's weight.

What's for Dinner?

Learn to cook.

Want to feel like an instant gourmet? Peel and slice a chilled cucumber. Toss it with some interesting vinegar. Take the time to plate it nicely. Top it with some nice Maldon salt. Bask in the compliments. Or just hog it all for yourself.

That just shows you how a little thought and care, and even minimal effort, can transform simple ingredients into a lovely meal. It's a small start, but it's a start.

If you don't cook already, learn how. I know that for many people it's a mysterious and fussy process. There are even men who have been poisoned into thinking that it's "a woman's job". It's actually everybody's job, and why should women get all the fun? Think of cooking as using fire and knives to turn ingredients into food. It really is fun, and often therapeutic.

I understand that there are times when we haven't the time nor energy to get fancy in the kitchen. But as you gain experience preparing food you'll learn to improvise, and find all kinds of quick and easy things you can do.

You already know to start with your veggie course. The suggestion to make one meal per day a big salad is a rather good one. And salads are a wonderful opportunity to improvise and feel like a fancy cook without having to actually do anything fancy. Or even actually *cook*.

Here's a master recipe for a lovely, filling salad:

1. Tear up and wash some leafy greens. (Invest in a good salad spinner.)
2. Chop up some fruits and vegetables that are either pre-cooked or that can be eaten raw.
3. Toss in a can of pre-cooked beans, or maybe chickpeas.
4. Make a dressing by whisking a little vinegar with some nice oil. Maybe some herbs, or even honey and mustard. (A good rule of thumb is 1 part vinegar to 3 parts oil.)
5. Toss.
6. Serve.

Really. *Cook's Illustrated* has said that a salad can be defined as "anything you put vinegar on", and I agree. I have yet to find flavors that don't go together wonderfully. Think about including sweet, sour, savory, and bitter for a broad flavor profile. It's like a roulette game that you can't lose.

Hey — here's a boss salad tip I learned from a book by Thomas Keller. If his name doesn't ring a bell, he's the chef behind restaurants such as *The French Laundry* and *Bouchon*, and who came up with the ratatouille recipe for the Pixar film of the same name.

Use a wooden salad bowl for best results. Make (or open the bottle of) your dressing, and pour it around the edges of the empty bowl. This will coat most of the bowl in dressing. Now dump the greens in the bowl and toss with a pair of tongs. That way the dressing will end up evenly distributed, and you won't have a frustrating puddle at the bottom of the bowl. Plus it just feels fancy when you do it.

The best way to learn anything is by doing it. Start by finding some simple recipes for things you like. Make them by following the recipe for the first few times. Pretty soon you'll grok how it works, and you'll be riffing on what's in the cookbook (or on the web page).

The best tip for home cooks, and something the pros do is: **Taste as you go**. This is a good opportunity to let you know that, when cooking at home, it's OK to use as much salt as you want. The way people end up with too much sodium in their diet is eating a large proportion of commercially-pre packaged foods. It's educational to check the labels on the food you buy for sodium content, especially if your doctor has suggested cutting down. But it's highly unlikely you'll get anywhere near that level at home even if you go kind of crazy with the salt shaker.

Which you won't, because you're tasting as you go. You'll end up with perfectly seasoned food and even more accolades.

Maybe take a class.

There are many cooking classes out there. It may be the area I live in, but most of the ones I've found are pretty expensive. Fortunately there's an on-line course that I took which is crazy cheap and really excellent. America's Test Kitchen, which sprang from Cook's Illustrated, has an online cooking school which lets you do as many lessons as you want for a flat monthly fee. If you're someone who eats out a lot because you don't know how to cook, it will pay for itself in the first month, and the quality of instruction is excellent. The URL is simple: www.onlinecookingschool.com. They will literally take you from boiling water (because simmering and boiling turn out to be two different things) through knife skills and on up to making dishes and desserts that will dazzle you, your family, and your guests. It's wicked fun.

Relax and Enjoy Your Food

I've saved some of the best news for last. If you enjoy your food, namely eat foods that you enjoy, you just might get more nutrition from it. A study done in the late 70's[5] on Swedish and Thai women found that more iron was absorbed from familiar, enjoyed foods than from each other's cuisines. Even more surprising, when the Thai women were given their exact same food, but blended to resemble baby food, there was less iron

---

[5] Hallberg et al. Tufts University Health & Nutrition Letter, October 2000

absorption. Now, all the usual caveats about a single study apply, of course. But there is a plausible mechanism of action. You've heard the expression that we first eat with our eyes. When the brain anticipates food it knows and loves it responds with more chemical preparation in the form of enzymes in saliva, gastric, pancreatic, and intestinal liquids. This is known as the cephalic phase of eating.

And even if the science for that assertion turns out to be weak, at very worst you will have enjoyed your food more. A government panel meeting in 1995 considered recommending the phrase "enjoy a variety of foods". Some spoilsports worried that people might interpret that to mean a variety of doughnuts or something, I guess, and it ended up as "*eat* a variety of foods". Well, I'm team enjoy.

Summing it up, here's most of what you need to know:

Enjoy a variety of foods, mostly plants, including plenty of fruits and vegetables, not too much or too little.

What you eat today doesn't matter. What you eat this month matters a lot. Think big picture.

Drink when you're thirsty, eat when you're hungry. (And then stop.)

Ignore any attempts to make you afraid of a food or an ingredient.

Any food can be part of a healthy diet. There are no junk foods.

Get regular exercise, plenty of good sleep, and all the appropriate vaccines. Don't smoke or do drugs. Consume as little alcohol as possible.

Never let anybody make you feel guilty about how, or how much, you eat.

Let what you eat be a source of joy, nutrition, and carnal pleasure.

In other words, **relax and enjoy your food**.

Acknowledgements

My heartfelt thanks to Sara Shopkow for helpful feedback and casting an editor's eye. Special thanks to "SkepDoc" Harriet A. Hall, MD for not only being an inspiration and role model, but providing much-needed fact checking. The incomparable Jeff Pidgeon provided the beautiful artwork for which I am most grateful.

Thanks also to the early readers, Frank Marcollo, Dr. Stuart Farri-mond, and Dan Handley for their feedback, and to Britt Hermes for her expertise.

But most of all my thanks to my daughter Catalina, the brave badass who conquered anorexia while becoming the best sounding board and cheerleader a writer could ever want.

About the Author

Craig Good spent thirty one years at Pixar (and Lucasfilm before that), and is now an Assistant Professor at the California College of the Arts. He's guest-hosted and written for the *Skeptoid* podcast, and has been a guest on *The Skeptics' Guide to the Universe*. He has wide-ranging interests that include food and science. When his daughter was diagnosed with anorexia he got an up close look at how important it is to have a healthy relationship with food. As the author of *Relax and Enjoy Your Food* he's put on his science communicator hat to untangle the myths that keep us anxious and less healthy than we could be.

Made in the USA
Monee, IL
17 October 2021